Mind Over Fork

Mind Over Fork

Escape Dieting To Find
The Healthy Lifestyle You Deserve

Rebecca Turner

Mojo Triangle Books™
An Imprint Of

SARTORIS
LITERARY
GROUP

A traditional publisher
with a non-traditional approach to publishing

Library of Congress Control Number 2015942124
The book contains the opinions and ideas of its
author. It is sold with the understanding that the
author and publisher are not engaged in rendering
medical, psychological or health personal
professional services in the book. The reader should
consult their medical, health or other competent
professionals before adopting any of the suggestions
in this book or drawing inferences from it. The
author and publisher disclaim all responsibility for
any liability, loss or risk incurred as a consequence
of the application of any of the contents of this
book.

SARTORIS LITERARY GROUP
Metro Jackson, Mississippi, USA
www.sartorisliterary.com

To my parents, thank you for unconditional love and untiring support, your expectation for me to always give my best has lead me to have the courage to try anything once, including authoring a book

CONTENTS

Part I

Part II

INTRODUCTION

"We repeat what we don't repair"—Christine Langley-Obaugh

Do you have a dysfunctional relationship with food?

Do you have a negative body image?

Are you a serial dieter, going from one dieting plan to another, sinking into depression when your efforts end in failure—as they always seem to do?

If you answered yes to any one of the above questions, you are the audience for this book

Mind Over Fork addresses those questions by offering a holistic approach to weight control and wellness that is focused on the discovery of one's personal truth.

Before going through my own personal journey of discovery with these issues, I worked with many consulting clients, hosted weight-loss groups, and taught countless basic nutrition classes. I did a lot of nutrition counseling to people hungry to finally nip dieting in the bud. I convincingly talked about macronutrients, optimizing the combinations of food groups on your plate, and getting enough fiber. Occasionally, I'd offer candid advice on emotional eating or sugar cravings, but sort of brushed over it without any depth.

Even though I was able to give a persuasive speech on nutrition science and write a killer diet plan, I was failing at igniting any true behavior change in the majority of my clients. Scratching my head, I just didn't understand why clients and audiences could leave a session with me on such an information high and never lose a pound, or not enough to matter, and rarely keep it off.

What happened to my clients once I was out of sight?

The missing link is so obvious to me now that I would like to take a moment and offer all past clients and weight loss participants over the past years a big fat apology! Forgive me for the years of missing the most valuable piece of your food struggles and for just tossing nutrition facts at your forehead.

Mind Over Fork is all about moving past the plate and into the heart of the problem. Every dieter has a story, and a story can be rewritten to shift the direction of the plot and help the person come out on top. It just takes a little bit of effort to understand the current plot and reorganize the chain of events.

As a peace offering, I feel it is necessary to share with you a piece of my personal story.

I'll never forget the moment it hit me that my quest for fitness and eating healthy was making me sick; my passion had become a problem. In my early 20's I became engaged to be married, an exciting time in a young woman's life. Unfortunately, I vividly remember becoming extremely anxious and terribly afraid of having to eat cake in front of a crowd. It sounds so silly, but there is nothing funny about the pain of being afraid of food. In that instant, it was clear that my preoccupation with an ideal weight and the perfect diet was not just a phase, but an unhealthy obsession.

My daily thoughts were consumed with how to make "good" food choices, and how to survive the day without making "bad" food choices. That compulsive desire to do well, make others proud, and obtain affirmations was present in all areas of my life. At night I would analyze the day and look for all the mistakes made, and devise ways to avoid any the next day. Not realizing that the perfect image we are subjected to every day through the media was just a digital illusion. I used the number on the scale and my pace per mile to measure my self-worth. To top it off, I felt isolated, fundamentally broken, and convinced no one could possibly understand how it felt to be that uncomfortable in their own skin.

It wasn't until I fully faced the scope of my negative thought and behavior patterns that I found the courage to dig deep and repair the real issues to avoid repeating the self-destructive cycle. It is sort of ironic how an extreme sport like marathon running could be a catalyst for change. Fatefully, falling in love with endurance sports also gave me a reason to admire and respect my body as an amazing instrument that needed to be well nourished and taken care of, or my performance would suffer. Food began to have a vital purpose, and was no longer just a necessary annoyance.

Not long after that realization, I reconnected to the stillness within while out on a long run, and that propelled my journey to what amounted to a spiritual awakening. Reclaiming my life and obtaining a healthy relationship with food was more challenging than a marathon, but more rewarding than any medal. Life transformation is a true marathon, not a sprint.

Although my story can be summed up in a few paragraphs, I didn't change overnight, and fighting the inner battle to be freed from old patterns of thought and condemnation darn near killed me. But, with anything in life, I am a fighter who once I'm committed to something, I wholeheartedly see it through to the end. Once I got a taste of what the power of *Mind Over Fork* could do when practiced daily, I was relentless to live from that place of peace.

I tell my story as an advocate for those struggling with their personal connection with food choices, and loving their self-image. The truth is no one is immune to the suffering that can come with having a negative body image or feeling out of control with their dietary intake. This book addresses how dysfunctional eating from over- to under-eating can be triggered by bullying of all kinds, unrealistic expectations set by oneself or others, or an authority figure, a lack of information about nutrition basics, or as a result of specific events.

But the good news is that recovery from a dysfunctional food and self-image relationship is obtainable. I'm a living example of what is possible when there is a caring support system that helps one realize they are worth more than a number, that food is not the enemy, and that true balanced and healthy living is something worth fighting for daily and above all, it is attainable.

I truly am grateful for all my past disappointments because they laid the foundation for the new level of health and wholeness I now enjoy.

There is a saying that you can't understand freedom until you've experienced prison. Prisons come in many forms. Mine was a mental prison, and my negative body-image held me just as captive as steel bars and a lock and key.

The thing that makes me the most joyful is I have the tools to raise my daughter to love herself, respect food, and navigate this pop-culture world without (hopefully) being captivated by its false messages. At least I am going to give it my best shot! And, if you will allow me, I am honored to share some tools, techniques, and food solutions with you.

My intention for this book is to share with you the strategies I've learned to apply that have positively shaped my relationship with food and self-image. I respect you as the type of person that wants to change the quality of your well being, and repair a dysfunctional relationship with food.

I really believe we all have the desire to be healthy and feel alive, taking in all life has to offer. But, for most of us in the modern world, those visions of healthy living have become shrouded in the frustrations of yo-yo dieting, quick fixes, dead-end diets, and the lack of willpower to maintain any good eating plan. Most give up the effort to even try.

I'm asking you to work one more time toward creating a balanced and healthy life.

What is Mind Over Fork?

Mind Over Fork is a way of thinking that helps to repair and restore a person's relationship with food, terminate the need to diet, and make obtaining a balanced and healthy life attainable. In other words, it's an understanding of how your mind expresses itself in your life and creates what you consider to be your connection with food and self-image. Finally, it guides you through the transition from a focus on food's negative influence on your self-image to achieving a healthy lifestyle and enjoying a more positive self-image.

By adapting the centuries-old technique of Mindfulness—a form of meditation first developed by Buddhist priests more than 2500 years ago and more currently adapted by some psychologists as a means of teaching stress reduction—and by utilizing the innovative study of nuero-linguistic programming (NLP), I have found ways to see past the plate and deal with the real problem.

Don't get overwhelmed by the term. NLP is simply the study of the relationship between language, the brain, and the body. This approach was developed by John

Frinder, who has a M.A. in psychology, and John Grinder, who has a Ph.D. in linguistics. Learning how you think can help you better change *what* you think, which will be your key to obtaining lasting change. I have learned a great deal from their approach to learning.

Together, we will dive "under the hood" of your own thoughts around food and work to adjust them to get the healthy results desired. You will learn to recognize destructive, self-sabotaging behavior patterns and make the how and why connection.

This book will show you how to develop the nutrition skills needed to live the healthiest life you want to live, in the most balanced way. You will learn to appreciate and enjoy healthy eating in contrast to forcing yourself to adhere to a diet plan.

The mindful exercises provided at the end of each chapter in Part One and the food solutions in Part Two are tailored for practical applications that work as tools that have the potential to change your life. These skills can help you manage your motivations to eat well, exercise, and reduce or remove other poor health habits. The strength of Mindful Meditation, according to the Mayo Clinic, is its focus on conscious awareness: "You can observe your thoughts and emotions, but let them pass without judgment."

I intend to go head-to-head and challenge the cause of your destructive relationship with food and body image, and improve your well-being. You are going to learn how to destroy the blocks and breakdown the walls that have held you back from maintaining good health. You are going to learn the incredible power of choices, beliefs, and mental associations.

Most importantly, you'll learn how you can begin to use these powers to develop a balanced and healthy lifestyle that best suits your own personal desires.

It won't be an easy road, but it will be well worth traveling. I know this first hand. Once I decided to take control of my life from the mind down, the results were infectious. You're probably already shaking your head and thinking this dietitian doesn't understand my problems. I'll accept your skepticism wholeheartedly and dare you to prove me wrong by giving this entire book an honest try.

Attention: This is not a diet

We live in a world obsessed with instant success: physically, professionally, and spiritually. Celebrities, supplement companies and the media have rebooted the idea of good health so that it's become unrecognizable. Headlines read, "How to lose 10 lbs. in 10 days," or "Skinny in Sixty Seconds" and on and on, claiming real results, real fast. Today a poisonous idea persists that you can and should be able to lose weight and get fit overnight.

In this line of thinking, skinny = healthy and happy. We have become impatient with the process, because we see that magic number on the scale as an end in itself. We tell ourselves that we can take a pill, omit foods, drink shakes, wear wraps, or detox our way to better health, happiness, and skinny jeans. We think we can do a strict dietary challenge and fix all our complex food issues in a short time.

In fact, more and more we think we're actually entitled to be fit and fabulous. But it's a seductive mirage that is very dangerous. There are no overnight tricks, diets, or supplements that lead to true health. Everything, including wellbeing, comes with a time invested cost.

Until the past few decades, most people who achieved good health and a tone physique followed the same basic path: a healthy eating plan and regular physical activity. It wasn't easy, and it was never meant to be. The discipline to stick to a long-term plan paid off with benefits, including low-chronic disease risk, retaining mobility, age defying skin, and strong mental agility.

Nothing saddens me more than working with a client and hearing the story of how they lost 10, 20, or 100-plus pounds to eventually gain it all back. Or, after taking the huge step to have some form of surgery, shifted their dysfunctional thinking to other destructive behaviors such as drug or alcohol abuse, compulsive shopping, or sex addition.

Too often, people get caught up in losing the weight they forget to learn anything valuable about true behavior change, balanced food choices, or realistic exercise along the way. And, once they reach that magic number they can't tell you "how" they got there.

So many times people get to their skinny dream too quickly and are simply not really ready for it. While their weight loss was in the fast lane, their behavior and awareness was still in the slow lane. While they were playing the game and swallowing pills, sipping shakes, and skipping meals, they didn't work on the mental aspects of healthy lifestyle.

Let this be your guidebook for nourishing and progressing in your mind, body, and spiritual health all at the same time, without compromising any one. Together, we can develop the competency that ultimately will enable you to succeed at achieving your ideal of healthy living. Trust the plan and invest the time in your mental development as much as your dietary patterns. There are no shortcuts, **this is not a diet book,** and I'm looking for committed enthusiasts, only.

A Word of Caution

If you have a serious eating disorder—particularly anorexia nervosa or bulimia nervosa—the suggestions presented in this book may be of little benefit to you. You will need to speak to a physician, who may refer you to a psychologist for evaluation and counseling.

What are the indications of a serious eating disorder?

According to the American Academy of Family Physicians, you should ask yourself the following questions:

1) Are you underweight, but tell others you are overweight even when they say you are skinny?

2) After eating food do you ever try to get rid of the food by making yourself vomit or by taking laxatives?

3) Do you use food to control your emotions—that is, do you eat because you are sad—and do you then gain weight and experience even more sadness over gaining the weight?

4) Do you spend a lot of time worrying about how

you look?

5) Do you spend a lot of time worrying about how 5) Have you stopped having periods even though you have not entered menopause?

6) Have you noticed fine hair growing on your body?

Yes answers to any of the above questions indicate the need for a consultation with a physician. If you are diagnosed with a serious eating disorder you may be treated with medications for anxiety and depression, and undergo counseling to change the behaviors that preceded the eating disorder.

No answers indicate you are a good candidate to benefit from this book.

An Easy Recipe: How to use this book

I'd like you to read the chapters in sequence because each chapter builds on the earlier ones. Of course, you can and should revisit any or all the chapters as often as needed to fine tune these skills. Remember, it has taken you a lifetime to get into this mental rut; I provide tools for authentic results, but even Olympic athletes practice daily.

The book is divided into two sections. First, we will focus on conquering the mind and uncovering how it is currently working against you. The mental exercises found at the end of each chapter offer the real tools that will help change you and will make you feel more confident about sticking to the food solutions to follow.

Part Two shifts gears and gets to the meat and potatoes of a healthy eating plan. Eating healthy doesn't have to be daunting or mentally draining with counting calories, stressing over grams and ounces; it's just not necessary. In fact, that mindset is the very reason many don't even care to give healthy eating a try. It appears too complicated, and no fun!

My philosophy is that you don't have to control every eating circumstance (it's impossible, I've tried), but you can approach every situation in the most balanced way. My goal is to make achieving *Mind Over Fork* easy and attainable so you can create a balanced and healthy lifestyle for a lifetime.

Staying connected with like-minded people to help give a hug and high five along the way is important. I highly encourage you to take this journey with a friend, co-worker, or church group.

If you enter into this book with an open heart, mind, and willingness to dig deep into the questions and exercises provided, you may not remember who you were when you began this journey. In fact, within weeks of tackling these mental strategies and food solutions head on, even your friends and family may notice the change in you.

As you integrate these techniques into how you think about your food choices over and over, they will become second nature. You become more aware of your thinking and diet decisions, you'll become your own personal expert and never feel helpless or hopeless in the grocery store, at a restaurant, social event, or after an emotionally draining day, ever again.

Just remember: This book is not intended to treat individuals who suffer from an eating disorder, psychiatric or other medical diagnoses related to eating or food.

Anyone who applies the techniques outlined in the book will have an opportunity to transform their relationship with food and achieve greater overall satisfaction.

Are you hungry for healthy? Let's get started!

Rebecca Turner

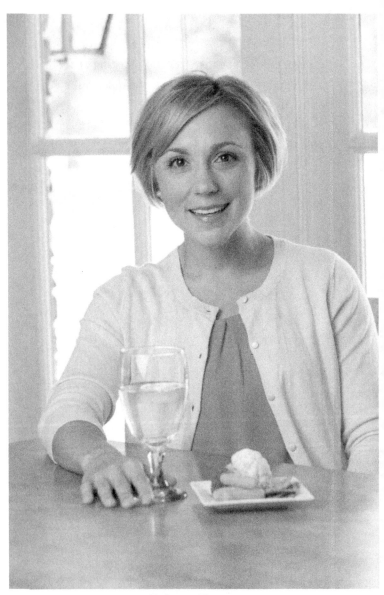

Rebecca Turner

Chapter 1
The Skinny on the Smoke Screen

"Change the way you look at things and the things you look at change" – Wayne W. Dyer

How do I look?

A question some people spend their lives asking others.

I can remember being a little girl getting dressed for Sunday service and anticipating a compliment on my outfit from my parents or grandparents. Once old enough to date and get married, I longed to feel attractive and even today, happily married, I always welcome a compliment on my appearance from my husband.

Who doesn't want to hear that they look younger than their actual age? I suppose it is just in our DNA. American culture has always been obsessed with youth. It began with our Founding Fathers, who put together one of the first youth movements in history. In 1776, James Madison was 25; Betsey Ross was 24; Alexander Hamilton was 21 and James Monroe was 18. They were only slightly older than the Beatles when they first came to America. Ever since the American Revolution, the battle has been on to remain forever young, fit, and trim.

Some cultures are obsessed with retaining youth with a focus on outward appearance and with endless varieties of hair dyes, wrinkle creams, and surgical procedures that attempt to delay aging.

You would have to be living under a rock with no internet access to not be aware of this mindset of striving for beauty, body image, a the willingness to use all means necessary to obtain superficial perfection. An ideal body is unattainable for the bulk of the planet's population, yet many ignore this reality. So, why do many allow a minority opinion to dictate their emotions, self-talk, and choices centered on food, apparel, or even a mate?

Simple, one's environment often helps to develop unrealistic expectations. Mainstream media, from advertising, magazines, television, and social networks spend lots of time and energy creating, maintaining, and engineering what I deem the "skinny smoke screen." They take advantage of the desire for results by offering products or services as the answer. The results are often disappointing for the consumer while profitable for the company.

Preying on the personal insecurities and fears of women, marketing agencies, corporations, and even small business boutiques have made millions, if not billions, by encouraging consumers to put faith into what they are selling as a way to obtain the image that is being portrayed as desirable. Over time, many buy into this smoke screen and develop unrealistic expectations to reach impossible standards of body perfection.

In real world warfare, a smoke screen, by definition is thick smoke released to mask the reality on the other side so enemy forces can take over without resistance. If only the skinny smoke screen was as visibly apparent as a big black cloud of dense smoke. The advertisement and marketing industry has become very successful using effective techniques to sell products and services. Understand that some consumers are vulnerable to the use of subtle and seductive messages that they need fixing, improving, or enhanced to be happy and healthy.

A successful advertising campaign convinces many that their products or services are needed to finally measure up. Slowly, over time many Westerners have become completely overtaken by this smoke screen and have lost touch with the reality that lies behind the mental decoy.

The skinny smoke screen distorts our view of healthy opinions and positive self-concepts. Often it doesn't allow us to see the person we really are. The truth is we were all born fundamentally faultless, adequate beings completely capable to eat till satisfaction, savor food and time, and thrive in the body size that was meant to best move us through this life.

Since this sinister smoke screen lies only within our individual mindsets, it often goes unrecognized and may continue to wreak havoc for a lifetime. If individuals could understand they hold the power to define their image and not be defined by the media or others, they could see that there was nothing wrong with striving to achieve their own natural figure.

A natural figure, assuming it is fed appropriate foods and engaged in ample physical activity, is always a worthy goal.

My prayer is that you awaken to the notion that most of your personal dislike of your body size, shape, or stature rest in your cooperation to continue to live on the wrong side of the smoke screen. I encourage you to start to question every product or service that claims to hold the key to getting you to the outward image of your dreams, as defined by others.

"*The body image of your dreams*" may be only a smoke screen. If every person on the planet had the identical height, weight, chest size, hair color, freckles, and long tamed hair, would that image hold the same luster and appeal? Would it hold any value?

It is healthy and perfectly normal to want to improve your health, nourish your body with quality food and engage in daily exercise. Even the desires to run a marathon, climb a mountain, or jump out of a plane can be considered healthy and normal.

But these worthy goals are often unmet or not sustained for life when the motivation is solely rooted in trying to become a perfect person that will be more loved and accepted based on your appearance or physical achievements.

In case you don't believe that good-hearted companies would use such devious techniques there is actually a term for it—puffery. According to *Merriam-Webster Dictionary*, puffery is an "exaggerated commendation especially for promotional purposes," also called "hype."

Puffery serves to "puff up" an exaggerated image of what is being described and is especially featured in testimonials. You know those captivating photos of lumpy, dumpy people in tight workout clothes next to a skinny and ripped version of themselves in another- puffery at its finest.   Every one of those types of promotions is captioned "not typical results," but few read those. Puffery is not illegal and is a very common method used in adverting.

If the claims made by puffery are false, how can they be legal? They can't be considered lies because no one can disprove them, nor prove them. A weight loss product can claim it is the best in the world, but no one can really prove that, nor disprove it, so the advertisement lives on.

Same goes for the best burger, car, or hair dyer—all puffery. However, advertisers cannot legally take their claims a step further and state the supplement or food contains ingredients that help prevent a specific ailment or disease because it is something science could prove or disprove.

See the deception and the grey line? Tell an audience a supplement prevents cancer would be a false claim, but calling it the best super food on the planet is legal and countless victims fall for it.

However, this use of exaggeration gets your attention and now their message is memorable. Enough run-ins with a memorable ad campaign and you will be clicking, purchasing, and consuming it before you realize it.

But don't think that the health and wellness or weight loss companies are the only ones using these well tested approaches to get you to purchase and consume. Fast and junk food corporations are all after your mighty dollar, too.

Ever seen an ad for a juicy hamburger or walked by a bakery and found you losing all sense of control and heading straight to the counter to place an order? That's not totally your lack of willpower.

All good marketers will try and entice each of the five senses to snag your limited attention to get you hook-line-and-sinker as a customer.

Have you ever wondered why some people totally fall for ridiculous puffery that you have no trouble seeing right through? For me, it's anything that promotes a cleansing or detox diet, I literally laugh-out-loud at the empty promises printed in bold on the box.

But I can be shopping on the same aisle with a friend, and they are totally checking out all the testimonials while I shake my head.

Within the last few years marketing experts have increased the use of celebrities and high profile physicians to endorse products. The ads are filled with puffery but the public is duped by the familiarity and perceived trustworthiness of the famous person.

I hope you begin to see that no one else shares your exact version of your life. Your mind chooses the smoke screens you will or will not believe in. Individual reality is a powerful filter that you created unintentionally over the course of your life.

Not every person falls for every deceptive smoke screen or puffery attempt, but each of us has our own triggers and areas of venerability. For some it is the fear of being seen as fat, for others it's being insecure with wrinkles, and some hope to prevent something as scary as cancer.

Many of us walk around with multiple hidden agendas that feed off the puffery claims. Wanting so badly to find the magic bullet primes many to hope this product really does perform as advertised, despite our own better judgment. And once our mind is engaged it triggers us to march straight to the checkout counter with some ridiculous product(s) while totally forgoing other options.

I am totally immune to unsubstantiated claims of popular cleansing systems, but I am still subject to falling prey to a smoke screen or two. Moving into my mid-thirties, with years spent bathing in the glorious sun, I'm secretly terrified of wrinkles and skin cancer. I'd be much more inclined to stop, read, and possibly buy into things that proclaim being able to help me avoid either.

Just stopping to be curious about the product and entertaining the shear possibility it could work continues to feed the scared piece of my soul.

Because you've chosen to read this book, you've probably already made a few attempts at dieting and weight loss. You've maybe worked on diet after diet and vigorously try to maintain a seat on the "diet wagon". However, I hope by now you are beginning to realize that our thoughts are a very powerful part of the process and continued success.

Many dieters are not aware of the tools that are available to them to deal with how they think and its effects on eating behavior, the foods they purchase, and why they fall off the wagon.

Don't be overwhelmed. The process I'm going to

immerse you in will offer new doors of possibilities.

The mind experiences life through sight, sound, touch, taste, and smell, but not everyone uses them all with the same intensity. When you take time to better understand
which of the five senses you're more sensitive to, it can be a powerful tool in moving forward with change.

Let's do our first mindful exercise designed to help you discover your inner preference.

Mindful Exercise:
Discovering Your Memory Bank

Think of the lunch you ate yesterday, or any particular meal that stood out from the day before. When you think of it, how are you seeing the meal? Is it still sitting in your refrigerator, spread out in front of you on a plate or napkin, or maybe it's half eaten? There are lots of ways you might recall yesterday's meals. Notice how you remembered it, first.

Next, examine how you are really seeing the meal. After all, it's not like the food just supernaturally appeared in front of you. Mentally take a good look at the image of the meal. See how your brain automatically retrieved data, created a mental picture and then your mind sort of said, "Yesterday's meal; here it is."

Remarkably, you lived through 24 hours yesterday, processing countless images of the day's events and encounters unaware that you would need this particular image until I requested you to call it up out of the mind to answer my question.

The main take away would be how did the image pop-up? Did you hear something, visually picture it, smell it, or remember the taste and texture? Whichever of the five senses you experienced first to recall yesterday's meal is likely your dominate sense related to food. For me, it's smell. I can stare at an ad about baked goods all day, but if I smell a bakery I will start tasting and dreaming of warm buttered bread.

Let's try another example. Think of a refrigerator you've had, whether you grew up in a house, an apartment, rented a home, or moved around a lot; there was some sort of refrigerator that stored food. Take notice of where your brain immediately went.

At the mention of a refrigerator an image popped up. Now, I bet you are vividly thinking of it, and can recall exactly how it looks. You see the color, the size, and you know whether it was a one or two handled door, with or without an icemaker. And, you know exactly how to open it.

You may be thinking, "Big deal, I just know it, after all I lived with it!" Being able to imagine your childhood refrigerator requires a new level of awareness. It takes slowing your thinking down and focusing on a specific frame of your lifetime movie.

Bring the image of your childhood refrigerator back up and let's open it and look inside. Can you recall the sound as the door opens? Does something clang that is magnetically attached to it? Is there a unique squeak to the hinge?

What about the strange sounds it makes in the middle

of night? Maybe you notice it often gets stuck or is too heavy for little hands to pull open. Think about the sensations that it evokes and how that helps keeps it in your memory.

Although it is just a refrigerator, you have lots of stored information about it that is recalled automatically. Of course you don't sit around most days and think of your childhood kitchen appliances, but when you are asked to recall it and you take time to remember it, you'll notice all the stored pictures, sounds, and sensations attached to this one object.

Now let's leave your childhood kitchen and think about the other refrigerators in your life, and imagine the differences. You'll have different images, thoughts, or emotions connected to the refrigerator at your grandparents, best friend's house, or even in the break room at the office. Each has its own unique collage of sensory attributes.

As you recall different situations and places, you may start to notice a variety of emotions attached to these memories. Take a moment and explore the images, thoughts, and emotions associated with something as simple as a refrigerator.

Reflecting on the emotional aspects of your memories, different refrigerators may evoke a range of feelings, from unpleasant because it was always empty, to neutral because you never really used it, to happy because some of your best meals came from the person who stocked it.

The desired take-away from this exercise is to better

understand that your associations, connections, and relationship with something as simple as a refrigerator are dictated by your unique experiences with the people, place, and atmosphere connected to each refrigerator.

Learning theory teaches that collectively all of our past personal experiences influence our current behavior. It is scary to realize that everything you have ever thought, felt, seen, heard, dreamed, or imagined has been sorted, categorized, and stored within the mind.

You can continue to test this theory with other random objects, or foods you have difficulty eating or refusing, and watch how your mind may start pulling up long forgotten images, sounds, feelings, taste, and smells from your personal memory inventory. For now, I just want you to be aware of how it all fits together.

***

Use this awareness exercise to your advantage to discover stored associations or memories that may be the root of faulty decisions making. Often food choices are determined by internal personal reality not by the outside world.

Just because a puffery advertisement touches a nerve and leaves you interested in buying into it doesn't mean you can't learn to respond differently. You just have to start making new memories to correspond to the circumstances.

Don't panic, we will discuss this all in future chapters. Right now, just take a big sigh of relief that an old dog can be taught new tricks!

When you better understand the relationship between

the mind and body you will be better equipped to take control. For many years mental health professionals have taught consumers that this mind-body relationship is closely tied to how our thoughts and feelings affect our brain chemistry. Approaches to change this brain chemistry range from using medication for a direct approach to using talk therapy designed to change thoughts and emotions, which also affect brain chemistry. The ideas presented in this book offer an eclectic approach to understanding and changing behavior.

The next time you feel stressed, happy, anxious, or sad your mind will recall a similar response once used to elevate or execrated a desired outcome and let your body know how to respond based on past patterns of behavior. In short, patterns of behavior get sharper with repeated memory visits.

Most of us act on memory cues unconsciously and without much effort. That is why it is so easy to whip through a drive through and the thought of passing it up literally weighs on your mind.

Or, how effortlessly you can go through the grocery store and come home with the same ole thing, because stopping to analyze and think about products that have no memory attached takes much more energy and effort.

And when you've had a hard day it's much easier to reach for the chardonnay, chips, or cookies that you have such sweet relaxing memories attached too then go for a run, grab an herbal tea, or take a hot bath that has no positive association linked to it yet.

Memories are highly personalized and rooted into our

everyday patterns of behavior; they don't change without resistance. In behavioral terms, you repeat behaviors that have been reinforced.

Learning to analyze one's thoughts and determine the connection to behavior are necessary in order to step through a smoke screen and obtain power over food choices that contribute to healthy living.

In the next few chapters you can learn to break down your thoughts and analyze why you keep repeating unhealthy behaviors. You will learn ways to increase power over your thoughts so you may achieve the outcomes you desire and maintain a healthy lifestyle. In brief, you will start learning to put mind over fork.

Chapter 2
Conquer Personal Communication

"Life consists of what a man is thinking of all day."
—Ralph Waldo Emerson

For those who have an unhealthy relationship with food special occasions such as weddings, birthdays, anniversaries, graduations, and vacations may create unavoidable stressful situations, especially for women.

Why? They require a "little black dress" or the equivalent that is a far cry from our causal and comfortable daily wardrobe. For me it never fails, those pesky body image issues hidden behind elastic pants will bubble straight to the surface every time I start to consider what to wear to an event or pack for a get-a-away.

Celebrations and trips most often come with some notice. Many who are body-image obsessed use this prep-time to shape up before sliding into that slinky dress or bathing suit.

Come on, if this is you, admit it, you've done it before, opened the invitation straight from the mailbox or immediately after booking the hotel, you instantly counted the days left to lose a few pounds, tone up, and create your ideal self.

The invitation goes on the refrigerator and life goes

on as normal. Suddenly you are standing in your closet the eve of the event face to face with that "little black dress" and wondering where did the prep-time go? The closet begins to close in around you as you stand there suffocating in body-image anxiety.

This is exactly what happened to me after I received my first wedding invitation after having my daughter. I looked at my dear friend's special day as my opportunity to get fit and fabulous on a deadline.

But life went on without any lifestyle changes. Inevitably I ended up standing in my closet having a meltdown about how lousy I was for allowing the time and opportunity to slip by.

My self-talk began badgering me for the fries I stole off my husband's plate, for the brownie enjoyed as a splurge, and for the exercise that was missed because life with a newborn is unpredictable. Without warning I was at war with myself, about myself, and I didn't stand a chance. I just kept letting the negative thoughts keep pouring in until I had literally made myself cry!

Truth is I had not set a good plan in motion to ignite any change, but the bigger issue at hand was all the negative self-conversation going on between my ears that would provide zero benefit but a lot of hard feelings. I had gotten into a terrible habit of self-shaming about my body for years and it was destructive.

Honestly, it had become a nightly ritual to lie in bed and replay all my food and behavior choices that day and pick out the bad ones and then scold myself. I was literally addicted to self-harming with my own words.

Similar to how someone tries to release pain by causing pain, I would use harmful self-talk to verbally abuse myself as a way to deal with the pain of disappointing myself. If I had to guess, I'd imagine I'm not alone. Some of you have been there, done that, and know exactly what I am talking about, too.

Don't be ashamed.

You may be a person who walks around with negative thoughts bombarding your mind. You may cleverly devise patterns of little nagging thoughts, suspicions, doubts, fears, wonderings, reasoning, and theories of why life isn't going as planned without realizing that this behavior sets up strongholds in your mind.

A stronghold is an area in which we are held in bondage (in prison) due to our way of thinking. Many who struggle to control their food choices or stick to a healthy eating plan do so because they have not learned to control their thoughts, first. They are simply unaware of how to accomplish more desirable thought patterns.

For many years I really believed that I was unhappy about my body image, life imperfections, and food struggles because I was not the person the world wanted or needed me to be or worthy of being happy with myself. And, certainly the Creator of the Universe wouldn't be pleased with anything less than perfect. Therefore, I felt like a huge disappointment all around.

I blamed my misery on my in ability to just do, say, or act in the "right way." If I could just make it through a day without one bite of "bad foods," saying a "bad word," making a "bad judgment," a "bad grade" or "bad impression" on anyone including myself, then, I thought, I would be happy. Somehow I was convinced I didn't deserve the get-out-jail-free-card I allowed others to have.

This went on for years. I finally faced the truth, which was that none of these perfect "doings" had to make me unhappy if I chose to have the right attitude and mindset about myself.

My thoughts were what made me miserable, not my perfect imperfections. I never received the joy, contentment, and happiness I desired until I realized, my actions and self-image where not the problem, I had some serious stinking thinking.

If you listened to a recording of what you said to yourself, about yourself, every day, how would you react? Even worse, what if that recording was played for all to hear? If you are horrified by this possibility, you are not alone and more importantly; you need to believe that you can learn to improve your self-talk.

Hopefully you wouldn't stay in a relationship where another person berated you, yet you may have grown accustom to badgering yourself and somehow justifying it.

Those thoughts and mental horror movies get played over and over in your head a million times or more over a period of years, or decades. This is why it is difficult to get healthy and automatically stick to major lifestyle changes over night. It is a painful process to face our inner faults and deal with them. Our thought and behavior patterns explain why most are unsuccessful at maintaining a healthy life, but it must not be used as an excuse to stay in bondage.

I need you to start accepting the idea that your outward behavior is only a result of your internal conversations. Everyone, whether aware of it or not, engage in endless self talk.

Often, we laugh when we see someone talking to themselves but we certainly do it, too. Chances are, you are reading these sentences and hearing your own voice talking in your head. Getting to know the muffled, yet demanding voice that echoes your every thought will position you to start taking control of the behaviors you desperately are trying to change.

There is a Proverb that states as a man thinks in his heart, so is he. According to the author of the book of Proverbs, thoughts are powerful and have creative ability. Many go through their day without realizing that the dialogue in their head is dictating the day's events.

Your thoughts are roadmaps for the universe. Every thought you have contributes to a positive or negative outcome. It is easy not to be concerned with some thoughts thinking they don't matter; besides no one else hears them. Personal thoughts create our individual world perspective.

To get the most out of this book you must understand that the quality of your overall well-being is determined by the quality of your self-communication.

You cannot have a positive, healthy life and a negative, unhealthy mind. Positive thinking is as vital to healthy living as a heartbeat and adequate blood pressure is vital to physical life.

It is easy to decide if your self-talk really needs

upgrading. The quality of any communication is judged according by the response it gets. If you're not getting the results that you have intend to achieve in the area of weight maintenance or exercise than it's a good chance you need to change your self-talk.

The Bible says that a tree is known by its fruit. If you are the tree then your thoughts are the seeds that dictate what kind of fruit you will bear.

Sticking with the theme of a tree, there is a story in India of a man who was told that there was a tree that could fulfill any desire, and naturally he went to search for it. The tradition of the legend believes that whoever happens to sit down for a moment under this tree will have his or her wish fulfilled; yet nobody knows where the tree is to be found. The kicker is the tree is the mind; its root is the heart.

If you spend your day saying you are unhealthy, unfit, unable, unmotivated, unworthy, exhausted, too busy, and sick and tired, it is likely you will develop a cycle of being sick and tired of life. I believe that problems with food and lifestyle changes are actually rooted in thinking patterns that actually produce the problems, the self-sabotaging, and presumed failures.

You may have a hard time believing that your thoughts manifest your reality. Think back over your life. All your possessions, career, lifestyle, and family structure started with a thought. Back in grade school you daydreamed, "Someday I should like to earn a degree, get married, own a home, have two kids, and drive a sports car."

At that time you had no money, no career, no capability; but the seed of thought was sown. Life goes on and perhaps years pass, but that seed has been working constantly throughout the entire universe to prepare you for that which you desired.

Of course life circumstances can easily derail a child's best-made dreams, but I'd guess that some of what you hoped for came to pass. If we could look back to all we have thought at the different stages of life, we would find that the line of fate or destiny was formed by a thought first. Thoughts prepare for us the happiness or unhappiness, or total well-being or total self-destruction which we experience.

Through self-reflection you probably can identify a time when your own thoughts and self-talk sabotaged a relationship or career choice or contributed to unnecessary sadness. Be easy on yourself, change it's easier said than done. Controlling the mind is like taming a ravaged, hungry beast.

There is hope, just because you're accustomed to counter-productive thinking, you don't have to accept it any longer. Once you become aware of the power of your thoughts, you are able to better arrange life to get the results you have desperately sought after, including a healthier lifestyle.

My hope is that as you become acquainted with the skills I've learned and applied in my own life, you will believe that you, too, can do this.

Now back to the example of the refrigerator in the previous exercise.

When I think of my mom's refrigerator I get fuzzy warm feelings because some my most favorite meals come from there and my relationship with my mom is special. Someone else could have done that very mindful exercise and instantly became anxious and overwhelmed with stress reliving their childhood memories of a simple refrigerator, especially if their relationship with their parents was strained and the empty frig was a lingering reminder that the family was in a struggle to survive.

Can you see how everyone's perceptions, even down to a cold box are vastly different?

By understanding this, you can truly begin to recognize your self-talk and inner battleground. This sets the stage for you to figure out how to give yourself more of what you do want and less of what you don't.

Starting today, one of the healthiest things you can do is become aware of how you are talking to yourself. It's ok if the words disappoint you, because this shows there is room for improvement. We can't fix what we aren't willing to face.

You can learn to take inventory of your thoughts. After you learn how to evaluate your thoughts, it's helpful to ask yourself, "What have I been thinking about today?"

The source of faulty thinking usually begins with outside influences. The key is how you assign emotions to those situations. Those emotions usually dictate your behavior.

We often experience our thoughts like we experience the weather. We accept and deal with whatever rolls in that day. "I just don't have time for breakfast... Today was hard; I'll treat myself to cookies.

One bite won't hurt … I want the burger so I might as well order the fries … No one expects me to really stick with this diet anyway… I don't like to exercise … I don't like vegetables. I look fat, feel fat, and I am just going to stay fat."

No matter what pops into their head they are at its mercy, never second guessing it and always agreeing with it and allowing it to manifest into unhealthy actions and painful self-regrets. Then with the regrets come more derogatory self-talk and the cycle continues.

There is certainly a better way to handle the negative atmosphere of your brain. An approach to tackling the battlefield of the mind is to remember how those thoughts are created. Every thought or feeling is created by stimuli.

The moment you touch, taste, smell, hear, or see something it is directed to the brain where it gets interpreted. Never forget we are sensory-based organisms programmed to respond.

Based on past memories and encounters with stimuli you assign a meaning to that sensation. This is why it is important for you to take time to analyze your thinking and begin to understand the connection.

For example, the smell and certainly the taste of coffee send happy signals all through my brain and body. I have definitely linked a positive reaction to all these coffee cues. Unlike the sound of my work phone dinging with a new email; often I cringe or get a "what now" mindset.

However, the sound of my daughter laughing or a hug from my husband can melt away the worst days lingering thoughts.

As you go through your day, you encounter stimuli that you assign or have already assigned meaning to it. Your thoughts produce emotions, and it's the emotions that generate your behavior. Just the thought of a cookie would be delicious right about now doesn't make you eat it, but that thought generates the pleasurable emotion you assigned to that double-chocolate-chunk the last time you ate it and so you cave in. Obviously, a thought is not a behavior but a thought drives emotions, which elicit behaviors.

It can be overwhelming to contemplate how you will be able to think about what you're thinking about, control it all and manage to make it through the day? The scope of this book is limited to an introduction of how thoughts and behaviors are related to eating.

First, pinpoint the behaviors you consider your biggest offenders: mindless eating, caving at restaurants, late night snacking, emotional cravings, or inability to choose broccoli over French fries.

Then try to go back to the thoughts and environmental factors that proceeded the behavior and evaluate the external input that triggered the emotion in the first place.

Take time to concentrate on your thoughts and allow yourself to visualize and engage your senses.

Think about the following statements:

"It's fun to go for ice-cream."

"I can relax with a glass of wine."

"That cookie ruined my whole diet today."

"I deserve a piece of chocolate."

"I can't live without coffee."

Despite how these emotions about food are stated, the real author of our feelings toward them is not the food itself. The real issues are the meanings we have assigned the food: fun, relaxing, deserving, life providing, and so on.

Bottom line: Stimulus to thought—thought to meaning—meaning to emotion—emotion to behavior. This entire cycle happens in an instant a billion times a day, and most often without our awareness. I encourage you to mark this day as the day you chose to commit to trying these new skills.

There are endless opportunities presented to us every day. In the beginning it will take your effort every day, every hour, and sometimes every meal to keep renewing your thinking. Remind yourself that it took many years to develop unhealthy thinking about food and the process of change takes time.

When you begin to feel that the battle of the mind is just too difficult and you aren't going to make it, then just choose to make one more health promoting thought before giving in. Bombarded with doubts and fears, we must take a stand with only one positive thought at a time.

"I can avoid this temptation this time."

"I will order water to drink at this meal."

"I will not go back for seconds this time."

"I will not buy the candy this time."

One positive thought, behavior, at a time.

Eating and drinking are daily activities with daily

temptations to go the unhealthy route. That is why it is important to choose health-generating thoughts. When we think healthy, we choose healthy.

When the battle seems endless and you think you'll never tame the tormenting thoughts, remember that you are reprogramming a very complicated system of thoughts, judgments, views, beliefs, opinions, and sensory-responses. Is it impossible? Not at all! Is it difficult? Heck yeah! But worth it.

Very often people ask, 'How long has one to go on this path to achieving mind over fork?' It only takes a moment to shift perception to value the part your mind plays in your happiness and health. But there is no limit to the length of this path. Staying on the path can be a lifelong process.

In my own life, I finally had to wake up and realize that I was living a health and wellness lie. On the outside I looked strong, fit, healthy, and put together. On the inside I was going to war every day with my thoughts and opinions of myself, body image, and overall value to this planet. I had many wrong mindsets and many mental strongholds that I had built up over years. And, it took me making up my mind that I would not quit and give up until I gained victory over my life and overall health.

The battle is yours to win, so stick with me.

Mindful Exercise:
Three people you need to forgive today

Your desire to expand past and finally conquer a negative relationship with food, distorted self-image, and a yearning for better quality of health has brought you to pick up this book. That tells me you are someone who values good health and wants more out of life.

No matter where you are right now on your wellness journey, you can rise higher, live healthier, and obtain an authentically balanced life.

I want you to know I enter this process with you with great respect. I may not speak to you face to face, but you have allowed me the privilege of sharing my story and this journey with you and I am deeply appreciative to have the opportunity to be your guide.

Before we go any further in this process together, I need you to take a moment and write down the age and weight that you were at your heaviest and lowest weights. Pause and reflect on those versions of you.

Next to each version write 2-3 sentences that best describes that version of you whether it is past or present. Next, write down your goal weight or pants/dress size or whatever numerical reference point that would make you feel validated once achieved.

Now, make a conscious decision to forgive each and every version of yourself. You may never find peace in this process nor be successful until you completely forgive and let go of the past with any perceived imperfections with any ns and failure. I encourage you to start this process with 100 percent self-compassion, otherwise you will likely nose-dive back into old habits. Only a clear and guilt free heart is ready to except new seeds to set root for a fresh start.

True forgiveness is giving up the idea the past can be different.

Forgive the heaviest you for the disappointments, for not getting with the program, for not being strong enough to tackle the issues, for not loving yourself enough to overcome the temptations around food.

Forgive the lowest weight you for not sticking with it, for validating to yourself and the world you couldn't do it, not worth the weight loss, and letting you believe that it might be possible.

Forgive the present and future you for regulating your worth and value and the ability to be happy on a goal weight or pants size. And most importantly go ahead and accept that no form of you in the future will ever do be perfect.

Forgiving yourself may seem silly, but is not. It is vital and the ultimate first step. Out loud, declare: I forgive me for letting myself down, giving into temptation, for disappointing myself and others."

Let's mark this milestone in thinking with shredding the paper to pieces as a symbol of forgiveness and those old wounds don't dictate your future.

One last thought to leave you with before we get to work. Most of you have tried a diet or two before which consisted of some form of "learning" about food and how to manipulate calorie intake to yield weight loss results. Do not destroy your motivation for learning something new by thinking you already know it!

Start this process with an open heart and mind. If you are willing to accept the challenge use the tools and techniques laid out in this book you can achieve a higher level of well-being.

Take a mindful moment to congratulate yourself; you've taken the first step to personal freedom from dieting and rebuilding your relationship with your self-image and food! So, hold every thought captive and discard any image that doesn't label you loved and valuable, gifted and able to accomplish goals that are within reach.

Chapter 3
Choices

"It is our choices, Harry, that show what we truly are, far more than our abilities." —
J.K. Rowling, Harry Potter and the Chamber of Secrets

I hear it all the time and I bet you have said it more than once, "I am so *ready* to lose this weight, get healthy, and be done with dieting!" And, it is fair to say that the proclamation of this readiness on multiple occasions is due to repeated unsuccessful attempts at making a lasting change. From eating healthier to being physically active or reducing time on social media, everyone has behaviors they'd like to gain control over.

As a registered dietitian, I find myself giving advice about changing ingrained unhealthy habits on a daily basis. Even though many are able to succeed in making desired changes in the *short term*, most fall victim to the original behavior patterns in the *long term*. What, then, does it mean to be "ready" to lose weight if it gets you nowhere?

Readiness is only the prerequisite for accomplishment. The two should not be confused! This is the first mistake. Just because you are "ready" does not mean you have accomplished your goal. It just means the pump is primed for work. The work itself is still yet to come.

Everyone who buys a new diet book, has a healthy

eating Pinterest board, or joins a gym has great intentions. But intentions are at best a compass leading you in the right direction. Good intentions won't buy or eat the wholesome foods, nor will it go the extra mile at the gym. It can only get you there. You can declare you'd like to run a marathon, but you'll need more than a desire to cross the finish line.

But don't be discouraged. Being ready is the first step, and the most important. Perhaps you have never thought about your eating behavior in terms of getting healthy or never thought about it seriously.

We think we are ready for change because we receive ideas about behavior or habits we might need to alter from others—family, doctors, and the media. The work necessary for maintaining successful healthy life choices is too difficult to be based solely on the suggestions of others. Motivation must be from within you.

I imagine since you picked up this book you have begun to actively think about the need to get healthy, to embrace what all that entitles, and give it a try. Here is where many get stuck; this stage of thinking can last anywhere from *a moment- to an entire lifetime.* My guess, if you have been stating you're "ready" to get healthy for years with no success, you are stuck in a rut *contemplating* the change.

What causes us to move from contemplation stage to success is a change in thinking and taking action through making choices with a defined purpose. Being unhealthy seems to be involuntary; something beyond your own control. The problem is you are trying to control a behavior without controlling the root.

You may believe that you are responsible for what you do, but not what you think. The truth is that you are fundamentally responsible for what you think, because it is only at this level that you can exercise the single agent for change; personal choice.

Working backwards, what you eat or drink originates with what you think, and then how you interpret those thoughts that dictate your actions. So much valuable time is lost doing food elimination challenges, sugar detoxes, and flirting with fad diets. Instead of waging another war on doughnuts, sodas, potatoes, and the couch, let's turn attention at what really bypasses the windows of opportunity, our daily choices.

Read this statement until you believe it: "I'm totally responsible for my general health and wellness. Every day I am co-creating with the universe to produce the wellness reality I live in." Repeat it until you feel a sense of belief and commitment.

If you are someone who believes that your circumstances are outside of your control and that you didn't choose this life, it chose you, then you may believe everything is left up to fate.

Think about it, if we have zero control over anything and are only subject to the randomness of circumstances then who is controlling it all? Sure, God Almighty is the author and creator of *all*, but even God gives us free will to choose! Having no choice or control over your life circumstances means slavery or robotic behavior. Having choices in any situation gives each of us the freedom to change and grow.

Life can deal unexpected blows, even in the health arena. For reasons beyond our understanding people who you would never expect get devastating health diagnoses, tragic events happen, and those who make healthy living choices can fall victim to a premature departure. While these types of headlines make the news, they are the exception and not the general rule.

According to the American Heart Association, about 600,000 people die of heart disease in the United States every year. That is one in every four deaths. Heart disease is the leading cause of death for both men and women, leaving families heartbroken and many lives cut short. Although there is often a genetic predisposition, lifestyle choices can help prevent or delay heart disease for the majority of us.

I wish the nightly news in every city across the Western world would pay respect and show the faces of every death that day due to preventable chronic disease: heart disease, diabetes, and high blood pressure. I am convinced it would shake people at the core to see the ridiculous number of lives lost every day to poor food choices and lack of ample physical activity.

I subscribe to the philosophy that I am a co-creator with the universe to produce my daily life and future events, including my health. I believe that an awakening to this concept can empower anyone, even those with many chronic health conditions. My hope is that people begin to understand that if they are not happy with their thoughts and behavior they have the power to change it.

Good health isn't an entitlement; but it is often a choice. It can be argued that much that is wrong with the world today is our collective sense of entitlement. In the weight-loss world, marketers have succeeded at convincing customers they are entitled to enjoy juice burgers, hot fries, milk shakes, and super-sized value on a daily basis, all while maintaining a desired weight.

Good health is a culmination of the choices you make every day. It is about the food you choose at the grocery store and the dessert you pass up. Good health is achieved by eating nutrient rich foods again and again and looking at broccoli as a privilege not a punishment. It's the temptation voice in your in head being overridden by the determination in your gut. It's about quenching your thirst for a healthier life by reaching for a glass of water.

It's about getting out the door and moving when the rest of the world is on the couch only dreaming about having the passion that you need to live each day healthy. It's about chasing the fatigue in a workout and not running from discomfort. It's about being surrounded by a crowd of peers and choosing the healthier road when there's not a single soul that affirms your good decision.

The good news is that seated in any restaurant are more and more people making difficult choices from beverages, to entrees, side items or whether or not to splurge, split or skip dessert. Their defined purpose is to enjoy their meal without sacrificing their health. You can choose that, too.

The mom with a defined purpose of feeding her family nutrient rich foods first will make difficult but healthy decisions, starting with making a grocery list that meets her family's health goals.

Every profession, including stay at home parenting, bears stresses or demanding responsibilities and schedules. Yet, in every profession there are people who excel at finding and working to maintain a balance that allows time for work, life, and physical activity. The person who makes the defined purpose to sneak in any extra movement will choose to take the stairs, park further away, or wear a pedometer and meet the steps goals, no matter. The decisions were made before getting out of bed.

Any action is a cause set in motion, whether you realize it or not. Every choice sends our health and life into a specific direction and every direction leads to a different outcome. A lifetime of poor food and inactivity choices will lead to a health crisis or chronic disease. Whereas after a period of time making proper food choices and physical activity points the way to life full of abundance, health, and opportunity.

If we really want to take control of our lives and health we must take control and responsibility of our choices. It isn't what we eat, drink or how we move once in a while that changes our health, but what we do consistently. One greasy meal won't make you unhealthy and one fiber rich vegetable meal won't make you healthy, either.

My entire life changed the day I made the commitment to choose a better way of thinking, living, and treating my body inside and out. Throughout college and early into my career I stated time and time again: I'd like to de-stress, kick the worry wheel, and learn to love myself, but it never made a lasting impact.

The problem was I had just been stating a preference and I hadn't made a committed decision with a defined purpose to start making different choices that would send my life into a different direction.

Understanding the transformation that comes with committed decision verses just stating a preference is a breakthrough in itself.

Where do you lie on the spectrum? Are you committed to health or is it still just a preference?

Be honest. Most of your New Year's resolutions to get healthy have just been you stating a preference, not a dedicated, no turning back, breaking point. Mentioned early, the intention of every resolution is good, but once the compass points the way, the traveler must take the steps towards the destination. Simply buying the airplane ticket won't get you out of town; you must board the plane and strap in.

Making a true decision cuts off any other possibility, when you truly decide to get healthy that's it, you never think about the possibility of falling off the wagon, again. No right-minded passenger tries to depart a commercial plane once it's left the ground. But many of us have weak decision-making skills in every area of life and haven't made a real decision in a long time.

When we don't consciously decide where we want to go on the journey of life we are left to be directed by the environment and not our own values, vision, or boundaries. We will explore values, vision, and boundaries in the next chapter.

For now understand that unless you select the destination and correct course as needed, you'll end up where ever the wind of circumstance takes you.

Unfortunately, it sometimes takes a huge wakeup call in the form of a health scare, chronic disease, and the realization that your own mortality is at stake before any true change happens. Yet even then some people never see the potential power that lies within their own decision-making.

In June don't worry with how you'll make it through the Holidays, just survive one meal at a time. When the Holidays begin don't worry with how many parties and temptations there will be from Halloween to New Year's Day, just focus on one day at a time.

Similar to any muscle, it takes repeated use to get stronger. Like the saying goes, marathons are accomplished one step, one mile at a time.

The instant you make a new choice about what foods to buy, cook, or eat you set in motion a new cause and effect in your life.

Formally stated, Newton's third law is: For every action, there is an equal and opposite reaction. Reflect back over your current and past choices with food and physical activity; are you pleased with the reaction caused by your actions, or lack of?

If you choose to take no new action, you will get no new results, and you haven't really committed to becoming a healthier version of yourself.

Remember, if you make a decision not to decide, you

have still made a decision.

Einstein defines insanity as doing the same thing over and over again and expecting different results. So, wouldn't you agree? Most of us continue to over eat, buy junk foods, slip through the drive-through and skip workouts all while crying out to a higher power, "Please help me loose a little weight and look better."

How can you tell if you are the cat that continues to chase its own tail while trying to catch a mouse? Simple, evaluate a typical weekday.

Most move through the week executing ingrained habits; some healthy, some not, but we continue to do them because it is just what we are use to.

You wake up too late to work out; skip breakfast because you skipped grocery shopping, which leads to not packing a lunch and pulling into the drive through. Afternoon comes and you desire a break from your desk. Instead of a brisk walk you head straight to the vending machine.

Later at home you become wrapped up in the kids' homework, laundry, and social media declaring that there is just not enough time, money, or support to be healthy. At night you prepare for bed telling yourself tomorrow you'll get on the wellness wagon. Tomorrow never comes becomes no new choices are ever made to break the cycle.

Why does it seem so difficult to do something as simple as eat right and move more? Let's face it, human beings like complexity. We don't want to take only one step; it is more interesting to look forward and contemplate multiple steps.

Sometimes a person who is seeking a healthier lifestyle can get caught up in all the possible routes and get stuck in a maze. This holds many back. The lure of complexity and the attempt to become educated in all the details can cause one to become paralyzed in making even the most simplistic, yet powerful healthy choices.

I am asking you to not complicate this process and stop worrying about mastering a degree in nutrition or physical activity before you jump on the wellness wagon for good. For the love of food and nutrition science, you don't need to understand the biochemistry of your macro- and micro- nutrients to get healthy.

Just start flipping switches and starting the engine and do the things you already know works! You don't even have to wait to finish this book to start making the healthier choices you knew all along would get you the results you desire most. Right now, name five things that would flip the healthy switch.

Over complicating making healthy choices is a major mental pitfall. A key element to succeeding at getting healthy or attaining any higher level of living is the ability to differentiate correctly between "I can't" and "I won't." As a rule, when someone truly "can't" do something, it's because he or she lacks the skill to do it; when somebody "won't" do something, it's because they lack the will to do it.

Personally, I can't dunk a basketball, fix a faulted light switch, rebuild an engine, or speak French. Equally, I won't cook without a recipe, run without a sports bra, put away my husband's work boots, or wear white after

Labor Day.

What are things you truly can't and won't do?

Though the distinction seems pretty clear, many dieters often say "I can't lose weight, find time to exercise, or eat healthy" when they actually mean "I won't." This simple substitute "I can't" for "I won't" lets many off the hook. Mentalities centered on "can't" become a one-step-solution used to put needed change on the back-burner for life. Therefore, in the mind of the individual he or she is not at fault for lack of progress.

As a nutrition expert, I am tickled at how people react the first time they dine out with me or invite me over for a meal. Holiday events are particularly humorous. More often than not, someone comments about their healthy or unhealthy choice or highlights the healthier items added to the menu in my honor.

It is amazing how quickly self-proclaimed incapable dieters know how to choose healthier foods when the nutritionist is sitting at the table.

This phenomenon often is referred to as the Hawthorne effect, also known as the observer effect. It occurs when individuals improve an aspect of their behavior in response to their awareness of being observed. In this case, people tend to eat better, or at minimum affirm their dietary downfalls when the food police are at the table.

If I had a dime every time I heard the following, I'd be rich and retired by now:

"I know I shouldn't order this."

"Look I got grilled over fried."

"Don't judge me on my soda; I just have to have it."

"I found this vegetable recipe I knew you would love."

"You order first, I want to see how you do it."

Usually I reassure companions I'm not judging them for their faulty food choices.

The reality is you don't need a dietitian to follow you around at every meal; you just need the awareness of your own tendency to conveniently mask your hypocrisy.

The word "can't" literally alters perspective about personal abilities. It assumes that the person lacks the resources to get the result desired, which in most cases, is not true at all.

Humans can be unbelievably resourceful when even slightly motivated. Many families figure out how to feed a household with wholesome foods on a tight budget. Working parents find time to squeeze in fitness for the whole family by letting go of screen time. Everyone can muster the courage to choose water to drink day in and day out without any hurdles.

The problem is, eventually you believe what you repeatedly tell yourself, whether it's true or not. Creativity gets drowned out and you lower your health expectations to meet the "I can't" standard you have set for yourself.

Often the things someone won't do are the things that would take them closer to where they pretend to be. We're all guilty of this in different areas of our life. Awareness is the first step to moving past distorted thinking.

Next time you feel like you can't choose healthy, no

matter the reason, just pretend a dietitian is standing right there with you: What would a dietitian approve of you eating or drinking?

Mindful Exercise:
The Pen is Mightier than the Pound

The American Journal of Preventive Medicine focused on the success of various weight-loss interventions and found that those who used a food journal an average of five days a week lost twice as much weight as those who did not. It makes good sense; writing down what you eat provides a foundation of personal accountability. Food journals force an increased awareness of eating habits and patterns. When used correctly it helps one spot dietary trends, pitfalls, and sneaky unhealthy behaviors.

If food journaling sounds overwhelming, it certainly doesn't have to be. Technology, websites, and apps have made it easier than ever to get detailed data of your diet, but it isn't necessary for this exercise to be a success. Simply find a system that works for you! Old school pen and paper does the trick and will keep you focused.

In fact, I recommend those serious about nipping dietary pitfalls in the bud to start with a small note book that would fit into a purse, daily planner, or easily carried. Find one that you can decorate or that speaks your own personality.

Like a diary you want it to be inviting and fun to go to and record. Ultimately the system you choose to track your food intake is up to you. The most important component of a food journal is that you use it!

Food journaling is simple: **If you bite it, write it!** That is as straight forward as I can describe it. Every meal, snack, and beverage should be noted for greatest awareness. If you are working with a dietitian or recording it for your doctor then try and track portion sizes, condiments, sauces, and cooking method to get a full dietary intake picture. It doesn't have to a complicated food entry to be an effective tool.

Here is a simple sketch of how a decent food journal could look like:

Breakfast
Time: _____
Mood: _____
Food: _____
Beverage: _____
Notes: _____

Repeat that style of entry for any snacks, lunch, and dinner. Since my approach is avoiding the need to have been over consumed with grams and ounces, you don't even have to add portion sizes if that overwhelms you.

Be sure to leave a box or section for each day to highlight those infamous BLTs: bites, licks, and taste. You'll be shocked at how they add up to significant calories or sugar intake.

Remember, if you bite it, write it and be honest with yourself. I can't help you help yourself if you aren't honest with yourself about what you bite, lick, taste, drink, or eat. Seriously, who wants to track every bite for a lifetime.

Not me, and you shouldn't have to either. The main intention of a food journal is to showcase areas that need improving with the understanding that you act upon the findings.

Nothing changes if nothing changes. Take time to look back and evaluate your food diary and highlight obvious mishaps like portion control, mindless snacking, or sugar overload. Then take that information and apply a healthier change to your very next meal.

In Part Two of this book we dive into conquering the fork. Your food journals will be imperative for you to know how your current habits stack up to my food solutions. Like a teacher with a red pen, I'll encourage you to evaluate your days, not as method of shaming you for your food choices, but to empower you to pinpoint what needs changing. I know food journals can be annoying, but while you are on this Mind Over Fork journey you should at the very least consistently keep a sketch of your daily intake.

To avoid major burnout or becoming obsessive with food entry just focus on journaling Monday through Friday or your traditional work week. Loosening the reins on the weekends allows for a little freedom to plan for next week and get a break, so that you can be back at it on Monday morning.

I cannot think of a better way to get a bird's eye view of your current choices and patterns of behavior than writing it all down for you to review. It may not even be as powerful as you had hoped the first few times you food journal and it may even be every discouraging to face how off track you are nutritionally, but don't give up on it.

Change is hard work and there are no quick fixes. Believe in the power of confronting your choices head on and keep on using it to better meal plan and reduce anxious shopping, cooking, eating, or choosing a healthier choice that your current habits want you to make.

Are you starting to see how you really do have all the resources you could ever want or need to begin?

Chapter 4

Vision

"Where there is no vision, the people perish."—
Proverbs 29:18 KJV

Alice came to a fork in the road.
'Which road do I take?' she asked.
'Where do you want to go?' responded the Cat.
'I don't know,' Alice answered.
'Then,' said the Cat, 'it *doesn't matter."*

There are many nuggets of empowering messages in
Alice in Wonderland, but this one rings so true- you will
never get to where you want to go if you don't know
where you want to go.

Imagine this. You walk into an airport and approach
the ticket counter and the staff member asks, "Where to?"
and you reply, "I don't want a ticket to Alaska." It sounds
silly and yet it's how many of us navigate getting healthy.
It is hard to succeed at a healthy lifestyle when all we are
concerned with is not being fat, chubby, or have cellulite.

If I sat down with you for a consultation, the first
question I would ask is, "What is your definition of
healthy?" Perhaps you've never pondered that question.
There is no definitive answer of what healthy is or should
look like for everyone on the planet. It's just not that
simple.

The online Webster Dictionary defines healthy as

having good health: not sick or injured. Well that isn't a very descriptive definition and leaves a lot to the imagination. To some, having good health is being physically active and competitive in sports such as running, triathlons, or league sports, as well as, being flexible enough to engage in yoga or Pilates. For others, it can be as simple as meeting the recommend steps daily or stretching in between conference calls at work.

There are those that make fresh, local, and organic foods a top priority and go to great lengths to stay within those boundaries to be healthy.

While others believe healthy eating can fall into an 80/20 rule of thumb where you focus on wholesome foods most of the time leaving room for caloric debauchery on occasion.

Farmer's market fresh, purely organic foods can be expensive and simply out of reach for many. Then there are multiple different dietary lifestyle choices: omnivores, paleo, pseudo-vegetarians, flexitarians, lacto-ovo vegetarians, pesco-vegetarians, vegetarians, vegans, and raw foodist to name a few.

None are 100 percent right or 100 percent wrong, and all clean eaters should unite to support farmers and sustainable agriculture.

Nonetheless, there are some people who do have to follow strict dietary guidelines to remain in good health, such as those suffering from celiac, lactose intolerance, and food allergies of all kinds. However, just because avoiding nutrients is vital to their health doesn't mean the same stands for the rest of us.

As you can see, agreeing on a definition of healthy is not easy. Get healthy, eat better, or move more are all good goals, but how that is defined for every individual is unique. Defining what healthy means to you is essential and nonnegotiable, if you ever want to keep this up for a lifetime. Besides, how are you going to make choices with a defined purpose as discussed in the previous chapter if you don't know the description for yourself?

Here is the clincher, you must be clear about the lifestyle you want to create, not just a number you want to reach on the scale. You have to set standards, firm boundaries, and values that are acceptable for yourself. If you are not clear on who you want to become, you'll find it is all too easy to slip back into patterns and attitudes of the past.

Together we will discover and develop the vision, values, and boundaries you should hold yourself accountable to. By the end of this chapter you will be on the road to your healthy ever after.

To get started you must know what you want: you need a vision. What's a healthy living vision? It's a lifestyle that you desire that foremost keeps you at a healthy weight, prevents or manages chronic disease, is achievable, appropriate, and most importantly, measurable. It is easy to mistake the skinny smokescreen for your vision. We can achieve goals defined as what you want easier than what you don't want.

If your goal is to achieve six packs abs, a thigh gap, or a sub 25-minute 5 k pace, this book doesn't address those goals but if you want to feel good in your own skin and be proud of your fitness accomplishments this book can help you.

Of all the thought-behavior techniques that helped me create an appropriate health and wellness vision for my life it was the Outcome Frame process that helped the most. The original version is structured to help in all areas of life, but I tweaked it to fit the very specific needs of eating better and moving more.

By using meditation and visualization of each goal you increase the likelihood of actually achieving it. Competitive athletes, scholars, musicians and performers are familiar with meditation and visualization exercises. The more frequently you visualize it, the clearer it becomes and with clarity you are better able to set into motion the steps towards that goal.

Therapists often use these techniques with people who are suffering with disabling health conditions and with patients who are trying to overcome fears, anxiety and numerous other emotional roadblocks. The origin is from antiquity but there are scores of professional groups who lay claim to their particular variation as the best.

First, think about your health and wellness vision, but feel free to apply these questions to any outcome you desire. A well-formed vision involves the following five questions, which were inspired by examples in *The Essential Guide to Neuro-Programing*, which we'll explore one at a time, using the sample vision of wanting to feel more energized, naturally.

1. What exactly do you want to achieve?

2. How will you know when you've achieved your vision?

3. What stops you from having your desired outcome already?

4. What resources will you need to help you create what you want?

5. What are the first five steps you need to take to achieve this result?

What exactly do you want to achieve?

Your vision should always be stated in positive terms and have a measureable outcome. Begin by visualizing what you want for your personal goal. What exactly does that goal look like? You must not be vague or have general vision/goals. Remember to use your senses to help you and be sure that you can actually measure your progress. Since it's always good to write things down, write your goal down and how you can determine if you are making progress. You can have several goals, so keep each one simple and very specific.

There is no right or wrong vision, but I recommend being cautious using numbers attached as the outcome. This journey is about so much more than numbers of any kind. Numbers are great tools to measure servings of vegetables, water ounces, or minutes exercised. Even numbers such as blood pressure, total cholesterol, or blood sugar are good to strive to improve. Those types of numbers can help you stay accountable and reach your overall goal. I'm specifically asking you not to use any number linked to pounds, inches, or pace per mile as a part of your vision.

Keep your vision positive—what you want, not what you don't want. Do not set goals of stopping this or that; instead, use the opposite of the negative thinking to positive alternatives. So, if you are tempted to set a goal to stop drinking sugary drinks consider the alternative such as increasing your consumption of water. The point of visualization is to see yourself doing what you want to achieve.

A snow skier never spends time visualizing a goal of not falling or not hitting the gates. They simply visualize or see in their mind's eye a win where they have bet their personal best time. They may spend hours and hours visualizing a series of steps such as getting in the blocks with confidence, breathing slowly, feeling the fresh cold air, and so forth.

Through meditation and using good visualization skills they experience multiple sensations associated with going quickly through the course, making every gate with great precision and speed.

Some good healthy lifestyle visions may be: *I'd like to eat a diet rich in whole foods. I'd like to be physically active most days of the week. I'd like to run a marathon, complete a triathlon, or conquer 10,000 steps daily. I'd like to learn to cook nutritious recipes. I'd like to get off certain medications. I'd like to control my diabetes with diet and exercise. I'd like to eat a plant-based diet. I'd like to support my local farmer's market. I'd like to grow a garden. I'd like to start a walking club at work.*

Vision concepts are truly limitless. Just keep them positive in nature.

It is interesting to note that the brain doesn't work well off negatives in general. If I told you not to think about sugar and caffeine, how do you not think of it? Every time you think, "I can't have sugar, I must avoid caffeine," you first have to think of sugary, caffeinated foods and beverages. Next, you must cast those images out and those thoughts probably provoked all types of sensory simulating pleasurable memories that you now have to fight off, too.

To get even more precise, if you set a goal of being more energetic, you will need to describe what having more energy means to you, using your senses. To do this, ask yourself, "What will I see, hear, or feel when I am feeling more energetic? Or, what might those around me notice if I were naturally more energetic?" Possible responses might be "When I'm feeling energetic, I'll feel like I'm really focused, that I'm fully present with whomever I am with or whichever task I'm working on. I'll be moving at a controlled pace, thinking clearly, easily able to make confident decisions about what to eat, drink, and work responsibilities. I'll approach each day renewed, and end each day with sincere gratitude for the quality, not quantity work that was accomplished."

It's important to not make your goal too broad that it becomes overwhelming. For example on the energetic vision/goal, you can narrow the focus a little so your vision becomes: "I want to feel more energetic at my job, at the gym, or with my family." Or, looking at one of the other examples it could be, "I want to eat a wholesome breakfast each day." "I'd like to conquer my first 5K."

Often we set a great goal, or vision for our life and forget to try it on for size, so to speak. It is unlikely that you can fully comprehend how truly satisfying it will really be until you have actually experienced the outcome.

To explore your vision of feeling more energetic, ask yourself, "What will feeling more energetic do for me at work? When I'm focused and thinking clearly, what else will that do for me that may be more important than just not feeling sluggish?"

A possible response might be, "When I'm focused, thinking clearly and making confident decisions, work will be of a higher quality in less amount of time.

I'll have the energy to notice the important task and the courage to side step the unnecessary fluff, freeing up more time. The less time I'm chained to a desk, the more time I have to take care of duties around the home.

When home chores are done more efficiently; I'd be less annoyed in the evenings when the family is home. Being less annoyed at my endless to-do list will leave me less stressed and more compassionate towards my family, lessening the chances of mommy guilt due to being short-tempered or easily frustrated with my family."

Taking time to actualize or try on your vision all the way to the end does more than just make you feel good. It's also a tool to make sure you don't choose a goal that might have unintended negative consequences leading you to fail because it's not worth the sacrifice it takes.

Case History

Shortly after getting engaged, Celeste bought a wonderful wedding dress. It was as if it was tailor made for her. It was stunning and fit like a glove. But there was a slight problem. Due to unforeseen circumstances, it turned out to be a pretty long engagement. Two years, if you can believe that.

Once the credit card had been swiped, a harmless comment was made by a bystander, "What happens if you gain weight between now and then?"

Celeste hadn't given that a second thought until that very moment. For the next two years she was obsessed with the question, "Will the dress still zip?"

For two years she was relentless with her diet and exercise. Never skipping a workout and always skipping dessert. Finally, on the day of her bachelorette party she snapped and sat on the floor in a friend's home, eating an entire pot of boxed macaroni and cheese declaring, "This is what happens when you deprive yourself for too long!"

There was tequila involved with that embarrassing episode and it got good laughs in her circle of friends. However, at the time she was emotionally drained from trying to walk the line of diet perfection for far too long.

Her intentions were good, but the unintended consequences about drove her mad.

It is much better to consider all of these consequences in advance. Be brutally honest with yourself if you are willing to do whatever it takes to reach your vision for a lifetime. Don't just think about suffering through until you reach that magic weight or measurement.

Make a mental movie of what life will be like five years from now once you've reached your vision.

Don't end up like Celeste. Don't reach a breaking point and snap because your vision is so unrealistic it takes any enjoyment out of your daily life.

I promise that is not a mental prison you ever want to voluntarily walk into. There is a happy medium for everyone looking to be healthy and enjoy all that life has to offer, including macaroni and cheese!

How will you know when you've achieved your vision?

Once you have pinpointed your vision down to the specifics using the first set of questions, you need to add some meat to the plan. This question requires you to create evidence that proves without a doubt that you've accomplished your goal or at minimum that you are making progress. Thinking through an appropriate timeline of confirmation and benchmarks will help you consider how soon, or how frequently you want to experience your vision. There is a relevant saying: a goal is a dream with a deadline.

Sure your vision maybe to run a marathon, but it's absurd to assume you could do it within a week! So when you contemplate, "How soon do I want to feel more energetic?" you may be tempted to answer, "Tomorrow!" A more realistic approach is to create a time frame that allows you to take the needed steps to cultivate authentic energy. However, it must be more concrete than a "someday" timeline.

To be effective, you might say, "I'd like to feel significantly more energetic within a month or two which will give you enough time to make lifestyle changes and come out of any withdrawals from current sugar and caffeine habits." To establish additional evidence, you could create benchmarks with your schedule, bed time, and sugar or caffeine intake.

What stops you from having your desired outcome already?

This question is crucial in revealing what you already know is the issue, plus the answers are where your action steps will be developed. Remember, you can't fix what you won't face and you'll always repeat what you don't repair.

When I ask myself what stops me from feeling more energetic, I immediately think, "I need a better schedule for work-life balance" and "I need to prioritize an electronic shut down and formal bedtime." Other thoughts are, "I rely on afternoon caffeine too much and tend to skip my late-day snack" and "I waste a lot of energy on meaningless tasks that aren't producing any positive result."

In addition, when I ask myself what stops me from feeling more energetic, I find myself feeling frustrated and thinking, "But I enjoy my afternoon cup of Joe and how do I choose which task are meaningless when I'm doing my best to do all I can to grow, promote, and engage my audience?" These thoughts are genuine, but limiting as they create an inner war that stops me from finding solutions. I need to take a step back and find the truth in my attachment to the causes of my problem.

The truth is what I'm currently doing isn't working and there is always a fine line between making things happen and letting them happen. More tasks don't equal more productivity.

Identifying real emotions tied to changing and processing through them creates a workable strategy for achieving your vision. Plus, it is more the experience of the coffee than the actual caffeine that I enjoy and I can find a way to keep it on some degree. I'll explain more about false associations in a following chapter.

What resources will you need to help you create what you want?

Now that you have created a to-do list of things that need to change you need to figure out if there are any resources you need to gather to execute the plan. Thinking through the resources list will make you aware of what you already have available that will contribute to the overall vision, plus any additional assets you need to invest in. Resources, in general, are knowledge, time, experience, money, contacts, support, equipment, electronics, or willpower.

You should ponder, "What resources do I have on hand right now that I can use to feel more energetic?"

Upon consideration, you might notice that nothing is

holding you back from an electronic shut down or formal bedtime other than a nonnegotiable boundary and little willpower. You can invest in a traditional alarm clock and leave your i-electronics in another room to charge overnight, lessening the temptation to check them before bed. You can set a nonnegotiable boundary not to consume caffeine after lunch and preplanning mid-day snacks for the week on Sundays.

To address the mindless time on social media you can turn off all notifications on your phone so you won't be spontaneously tempted to check it losing precious mental energy and physical time. Lastly, you can start making a tally of your entire daily and weekly task. Then go through each, assessing them for effectiveness and if the return is worth the time investment. With great conviction you must hold yourself accountable for no longer engaging in tasks that don't benefit your energy level any longer.

After taking time to examine all that it will take to generate more energy naturally, you may be surprised to see that you have everything you need already, minus a cheap alarm clock.

When you search through this question you may find that taking a cooking, gardening, or meal planning class would be a huge benefit. Or, you may discover investing in kitchen equipment such as inside grills, steamers, or quality knives to help you better prepare meals that you desire to eat. It could be a new pair of gym shoes, sports bras, or a few personal training sessions to better understand weights.

If you find you don't have the financial backing to

generate all the resources you desire, make two columns for now and later. Then use those that cost money as rewards or goals in themselves to save up for and look forward too. I promise you have more resources already on hand to get healthy than you realize and under no circumstances should you put off making a change until you have all the resources you desire.

What are the first five steps you need to take to achieve this result?

Without action, a goal is just an idea. Going back to the timeline I created of seeing a positive shift in energy within 4-6 weeks, I will want to insert at minimum five measurable action steps to help ensure results.

Doing this helps to break who, what, when, and where into manageable bite sized pieces. You should also be able to evaluate benchmarks with a simple yes or no.

Below are five specific action steps to take within 4-6 weeks.

• Purchase a traditional alarm clock and let electronics charge overnight in the kitchen.
• Use your smart phone only for calls
• Only drink and eat non-caffeine after lunch
• Preplan and prepare a healthy afternoon snacks for the week.
• Create a list of all daily and weekly tasks and evaluate effectiveness.

Notice how you can easily and efficiently evaluate whether you accomplished each action step with a yes or no. Did you purchase an alarm clock and remove your electronics from the bedroom? It's either yes or no. Are notifications for social media and email still on my phone? It's a simple yes or no.

Others could be, "Did I preplan my meals this week? Did I go to the local farmer's market at least once a month? Did I walk 10,000 steps, today?" All action steps can be evaluated with a yes or no, leaving no grey area.

It will obviously take a bit of willpower to employ your action steps, but it is a lot easier to accomplish tasks that have been well thought out, with a concise timeline, that is based on a clear well-formed vision.

Mindful Exercise: Create a Vision Board

To better understand the vision for your future health and life I want you to spend time creating an actual vision board. It is a simple exercise that can help you realize the health and wellness lifestyle of your dreams into reality.

What is it? A vision board is a simple visual representation or collage of the things that you want to have, be, or do in your life. It can be pictures, quotes, scratch ideas, hand drawings, or whatever catches your attention that represents a goal, dream, or wish. Always keeping your eyes, ears, and attention open to whatever grabs or your attention and sparks your heart's desire.

You can use a poster board, designate a notebook, a napkin, or even a Pinterest board. The point and purpose of a vision board is to put your image of success directly in front of you where you can see it often, if not daily. I want you to have it in view so that you constantly think about it, envision it, and meditate on it daily.

By being on the lookout for pictures, quotes, or writings that charge your emotions with passion, you will notice you will begin to manifest those things into your life.

It's really quite amazing how it works and what a positive, uplifting experience it is to daydream about the life you want and then see it start to all come together. If nothing else, the exercise will help you better develop a solid idea of what healthy means to you.

Obviously, you can have a vision board for a broad spectrum of things in life, but here we are focusing on your vision for your health and wellness. I suggest an 8x10 card stock to start (or Pinterest) and locate what "healthy" looks like for you. There only one rule: You can NOT focus on specific body images or body parts.

Cut out (or pin) healthy meals that you would realistically eat, families exercising together, a certain marathon or 5k race you want to accomplish. Look for words that inspire you like stronger, faster, well rested, and nourished. Locate quotes that uplift you and say all the right things.

It could be places you want to run, bike, swim, or mountains you dream to climb. Maybe it is a normal blood pressure, blood sugar, or cholesterol, or cancer free report. Find those positive numbers and add them to the board.

Don't leave out skills you want to develop such as healthy cooking, yoga, or ice skating. This is not complicated; it's empowering and setting the stage to significantly change your entire well-being. No two vision boards will be the same, because no two visions of healthy are the same.

Now start collecting and fantasizing. Leave logic out of the equation. If the sky were the limits, what does a healthy lifestyle would look like for you.

Chapter 5

No Fear, No Failure

"I have not failed. I've just found 10,000 ways that won't work."--Thomas A. Edison

If I posed the question—"What are you afraid of?"—you would probably be able to spout off things such as spiders, snakes, the dark, or ticks. Confession: those are just my unimportant terrors, but you may also say speaking in public, germs, or a countless other things.

Fear is no laughing matter. It would do all some good to dig deep to understand our utmost fears in order to move beyond them.

The *Webster Dictionary* defines fear as a distressing emotion aroused by impending danger, whether the threat is real or imagined.

I argue a true fear is much more than a goose-bump or feeling; it is the paralyzing force that keeps one stuck in the mud of misery. Don't be fooled. Fear has many faces masquerading throughout our daily life as nervousness, dread, anxiety, or overeating.

It is my opinion that to break any pattern of unhealthy behavior; whether it is smoking, binge eating, being a couch potato, or too much social media, one must first overcome a fear attached to the change itself. Fear is a mental stronghold that holds one back from mustering up the nerve to even try to change.

Fear is also often the spark that leads to self-sabotage. Fear can be a verb, an adjective, and a noun, a tangible obstacle standing in one's way of stepping into a higher level of being.

There are plenty of fears that can weigh a person down. When it comes to weight management and wellbeing most can be generalized into five categories: fear of people, fear of the unknown, fear of hunger, and fear of success or failure.

Fear of people sounds ridiculous unless they are approaching us to do harm. But harm happens in many different forms other than being held at gun point. When we experience deep hurt by another human-being we can build emotional and sometimes physical barriers for a sense of protection.

Many people who have been abused sexually, physically, verbally, or emotionally will carry invisible scars for a lifetime. Being overweight or obese can be an unconscious barricade to ever being hurt again.

These victims may start to lose weight, feel great, and then the moment other people offer positive compliments their inner scars flare up and they self-sabotage to stay hidden and out of sight. Staying out of sight or unattractive is a tactic to stay safe from potential harm. Keeping on the weight is a tool to keep people at a distance and a way to make sure true intimacy never has to happen.

Fear of the unknown will keep unhealthy, hurting, miserable people infinitely trapped in a destructive lifestyle. Social workers can tell tales of children who against all logic beg to stay with abusive caregivers. Those children have learned coping mechanisms to survive in this environment, regardless of how cruel their parents or foster parents may be.

The anxiety with not knowing what to expect can be more overwhelming than walking away from a clearly negative atmosphere. The same response can apply to women who live with abusive partners.

Let's face it, even though you are clearly fed up with being overweight, unhealthy, or simply unhappy with your overall well-being you are comfortable in the lifestyle, even if it's over-the-top chaotic.

Each of us has created a routine of habits that help us survive our day-to-day lives. Those mundane habits are so engrained it takes very little mental or physical effort to execute the same decisions over and over again.

For the most part, many of our errands and customs are done mindlessly. We shop for groceries, order off a menu, mindlessly snack, go back for seconds, and bypass the water as if it were on autopilot.

The truth is letting go of the familiar is terrifying and leaves us to wonder if we will even like the alternative. The idea that the grass isn't always greener on the other side is true, but we can't even get over the fear that we would have to leave our grass patch to even try out another!

Our thoughts and perceptions about the unknown can grow into a horror movie within minutes. Before we know it we have convinced ourselves that our current way of living is the only guaranteed way you'll stay content.

Case History

Bobbie is a grown woman who is afraid of the dark. Sadly, it has been her secret for as long as she can remember. Something about the unnerving stillness of the night, and all the creepy possibilities planted in her head from television and horror movies that make what should be the most relaxing, rejuvenating part of the day a literal nightmare.

It is as if when the lights go out and she can't "see," her other senses go into overdrive. She can literally smell, feel, and hear a pin drop. She hangs onto every sound and clings to her pillow as if it were a ledge on a high cliff. Of course, that makes it impossible to get much needed rest. It is a viscous cycle that she constantly works to overcome.

She is not 100 percent sure why letting her mind and body stop to recharge is such a problem, but those random sounds she hears at night amplify to the point where she develops a distorted fear of what is out there that she can't control. It is all about the unknown factors in her life.

During the daytime she is a rock star at organizing, planning, preparing, and prepping for the entire if's, and's, and but's that might, could, or should happen. She can sense a fire from a mile away and put it out before it becomes an issue. It is the nature of her job and the lifestyle she has become accustomed to.

The idea of not being in control of what happens while her mind is not on guard gives her chills. So, a false sense of security is to lie awake and wait for what probably will never transpire to happen. If a *zombie apocalypse did come, she would want to be the first in the family to scream!*

* * *

What Bobbie has yet to learn is that often our biggest monsters or bumps in the night are just a fear of the unknown, or the lack of being able to control whatever pops into view. In fact, fear and worry are first cousins. My all-time favorite explanation of worry is: "we are just *afraid* we won't get what we want." We worry and wait, while staying painstakingly afraid that the outcome won't be how we want it to be. Isn't that the truth?

Sadly someone who struggles to lose weight, eat healthy, get physically active, quit smoking, stop spending money, or any other negative behavior you pray to get a grip on might notice that you are just terrified of what life will be like "without" chips, couch time, cigarettes, new shoes, or that "it."

We stay focused on what we are "loosing" versus potentially "gaining". Your comfort may dwell in what is predictable and fear accompanies change, often viewed as the unknown.

Uncertainty can be terrifying. But Deepak Chopra reminds us there is no evolution where there is no uncertainty. You cannot step into the next level of blessings the Universe has for you if you choose to remain stagnate in your comfort zone. And, quite frankly not all comfort zones are comfortable.

Not sleeping, is not comfortable! Having a negative relationship with food is not comfortable! The consequences of staying overweight just to be unseen are not comfortable!

Even if it is hard, I bet you can agree with me that in some capacity you are using weight as a physical barrier to the rest of the world and that the fear of the unknown is likely part of your battle. What you may not think of as a real issue or true anxiety is the potential fear of hunger.

Let me explain.

Reflect back over your lifespan to this point. Have you ever experience a time of painful lack, such as a shortage of affection or vital resources for survival: food, water, or shelter.

A person who has the good fortune of not knowing true shortage of any kind can get a hunger twinge and keep on about the day knowing eventually they will stop to eat.

Someone who grew up in a food insecure home, meaning there were times that there wasn't enough food to go around or no food at all, may have an adverse reaction to the feeling of hunger.

Also those who have an emotionally or physically absent parent or spouse may unconsciously be terrified of becoming hungry because it triggers hidden painful emotions of not being fulfilled in one area of life so they unconsciously fill-up in another.

Unintentionally, one will mindlessly eat, snack a lot, or do anything in their power to avoid becoming or experiencing hunger. Another tell-tell sign of fear of lack or hunger would be to peak into your pantry, cabinets, or freezer. With the exception a well-planned emergency food kit, is there enough food to last months and months?

Do you store multiple cans of the same food, snack, condiment, or frozen meals only to replace the surplus every time one is used? For example, do you have three to five bottles of ketchup and replace one every time it is used even though there are still multiple available for use? Or have five or more cans of the same food like tomatoes or beans but only use a can every once in a while and then replace it immediately.

Perhaps you are simply conscious of the problems you would face if a natural disaster—tornado, hurricane, snow storm, flood, etc.—hit and left you unable to leave your house for food and water.

Unfortunately, for some families living with food insecurity, not knowing if they will always have enough to eat is not a fear but a reality. They live in a vicious cycle of feast and famine.

When food is available they feast away trying to satisfy that deep rooted hunger felt during the famine that is sure to come, when food isn't readily available.

Emotionally this is a draining and damaging state to live in, but it also puts a strain on a person's metabolism. Our bodies are wonderfully made to protect and preserve life and will slow down the metabolism and store on to calories during the feasting period because it knows through experience that a famine is likely to be coming. This is one way we have the paradox of being overweight yet undernourished and hungry.

Another eye-opening fear that maybe troubling your

efforts to obtain the healthy life you claim to want, is the fear of success. But success is what everyone is after so who would be afraid of it? Plenty of people for lots of reasons.

I'd place bets that you have a lot riding on your life after weight loss. You've daydreamed that you will be happier, find friends, hobbies, attract a mate, or get a raise once the weight is off. All your unhappiness lies in you not being fit, fabulous, and forty pounds lighter.

For years, or decades you have used your weight or your struggle with weight loss as a scapegoat to all your woes in life. So, what happens if you did succeed and achieved a healthy weight and heaven forbidden still don't feel validated? What if the lighter version of you doesn't bring you the happiness you dreamed about? What will you use as your blame for all the other emotional baggage you carry daily?

It sounds cruel to even accuse someone of keeping weight on to stay in their victim mentality. But that is exactly what I am saying that some people do, and often without even being aware of it.

This fear of success also plays into the fear of the unknown. What will work, dating, or your marriage be like if you look, eat, shop, and live completely differently than today? That is scary stuff to contemplate.

In all honesty, I have dreamt of being a strong athlete and standing tall in my own short skin. The idea of letting nature carve out the figure I was meant to have with a little weight lifting and pushing the limits in fitness has always excited and scared me. I've daydreamed of being able to dead lift, back squat, do pull-ups and climb ropes like a ninja.

I've had these hidden physical fitness dreams since college, but never pursued them out of fear of getting "bulky" or looking "manly" or having big arms or thighs. My arms and thighs have always been on the bigger by nature side. Not huge, but no thigh gap here! I was self-conscious of not having the slender shoulders and arms that looked great in a tank top, so I did light weights, high cardio to keep as thin as possible.

I was terrified of the unknown that came with surrendering to my deepest desires.

Thankfully, I am on a different journey as I write these words of finally attempting the types of exercise I've always dreamt of conquering. The first five pounds of muscle I gained made my stomach sink and skin itch, but I have made a committed decision to see this process through for a year.

The exhilarating feelings that comes from conquering a fear and doing a pull-up far outweighs the false sense of protection that came with a superficial number on the scale.

So, like many of you, I still struggle with fears of success and change.

Finally, the most universal distress of them all that embodies all the above doubts and more is the fear of failure. The idea of disappointing someone, being disappointed, or missing the mark can be so paralyzing that sitting still feels safer than taking the slightest step.

Have you ever felt like a failure at being healthy

because you slept in instead of worked out, overindulged in festive temptations, or allowed the lure of a drive-thru to override the nutritious option at home?

On the flip side, have you ever felt like being healthy isn't so hard after you logged in miles, ordered a water, and managed to cook a nutritious meal from scratch?

Too often we get caught up in self-condemning every single unhealthy choice and self-praising the healthy ones that we lose sight of the bigger picture.

Our self-confidence in living a healthy life should never be built on the unpredictability of each day or in the fate of one wrong or right choice. It's true we are in complete control of the choices we make and should live with an intention to always choose the healthier path, daily. Where we get sidelined is labeling any unhealthy choice as a failure.

I believe there is no such thing as failure in life, only outcomes. Obviously, not every result is positive or helpful to the cause of healthy living and there are always consequences attached to our choices.

Over sleeping and missing a workout, overeating chocolate, and getting meals through a window won't help you cultivate good health, but each decision provides you with tangible evidence you can use to evaluate the outcome.

Knowing that skipping workouts, eating too many treats, and choosing fast foods, leaves you sluggish, bloated, and disappointed, can become the leverage you need to push past the next temptation and make a healthier choice. Becoming keenly aware that staying hydrated with water, eating a plant based diet, and moving regularly, leaves you feeling alive, in control, and well nourished, can certainly be the motivating factors that keep you coming back for more.

What matters is that you notice when your choices don't provide the results you want, and you consciously decide to try a different approach the next time. Sometimes it takes a few greasy, sugary, or deep-fried choices to remind us why we committed to a healthier life in the first place. And, at times those foods are rightfully savored because we know the choice isn't a failure, it's a decision to responsibly eat foods we fully understand can't be the norm.

By living each day with a goal for healthy living creating a healthy lifestyle will not require constant self-assessment if our choices are providing desired results. It's a process of changing your thoughts about the function of food.

Cease labeling decisions during the process as a failure or success. They are mere outcomes. And see the process of obtaining good health as an ongoing opportunity to become your own life coach with an eye on the reward of true health.

Do not invite the idea of being a failure into you're your daily life. Simply stay alert and recognize the internal signals that provide a sense of direction to the healthiest choices, and you'll be sure to find your own way. Focus on learning to create internal signals for yourself.

Unfortunately, some adults forget about the

fearlessness they were born with and stop looking for creative ways to solve obstacles. They simply try once, maybe twice, and then declare that healthy living just isn't for them or this is the best I can do. Sadly, when we spend time chasing every diet and exercise program the results are often disappointing.

What will work for you may take time and effort to discover. However, if the goal is focused on developing and maintaining a healthy lifestyle rather than weight or size, success is much more likely and weight and size will usually follow.

Remember to ask yourself: How do you plan to get healthy?

Don't shy away from broaching the issue one more time, but in a new and positive way. Your plan to get healthy may require you going to the edge of your comfort zone and trying something new.

That may feel scary but once you experience how it feels to stand toe-to-toe with a hurdle, leap over it, and survive, you'll begin to see that roadblocks are resolved by leaning into your ability to create solutions, not retract from it.

Michelangelo once said, "If people knew how hard I work, they wouldn't find my achievements so remarkable." Some attribute fitness or good health to ease, heredity, or a privilege, when in fact for the majority it's from great effort.

Today, tap into your innate persistence to achieve and get creative with multiple solutions to attainment better health. Go to the edge willingly and dare to see if there is an approach to finally kicking your fears, soda habit, getting off the couch, or allotting part of your grocery budget to more wholesome foods that you haven't tried yet. As Einstein said, no problem was ever solved from within the frame of thought that created the problem in the first place. Get excited about the action steps you have determined are necessary to achieve your healthy lifestyle.

The advantage you have each morning is having the outcome of yesterday to go by. If you didn't like your choices or how the day flowed then simply change your approach to get the outcome you want. If that approach doesn't work, then try another approach, until you find the path that works for you. Removing the idea of failure from your brain offers you the opportunity to keep trying until you choose a healthier path. Remind yourself that success breeds success.

I understand that you want the change to happen now, acquire instant results, and ready to move past unhealthy habits leaving them in the dust behind you. While your passion for success is great, I want you to fully accept the truth that renewing your current thinking to achieve mind over fork will take place little by little. Please, do not be discouraged if progress seems slow at first.

Everyone on any journey to obtain a positive shift in their life will have setbacks, you included.

Here are a few quotes for combating failure fatigue.

"I have not failed. I've just found 10,000 ways that won't work."—Thomas A. Edison

"I can accept failure, everyone fails at something. But I can't accept not trying."—Michael Jordan

"Sometimes by losing a battle you find a new way to win the war."—Donald Trump

Perhaps your brain and body are screaming, "I'm not going to get healthy; this is too hard. I always fail, I never stick with it, and nothing ever changes. I'm sure other people don't have this much trouble eating the right foods and exercising. I may as well give up and eat whatever. I'm tired of trying. I try to do right, but it seems the world is stacked against me. Gosh, I'm just so disappointed in the way I eat."

Never forget, you become what you think. Think discouraging thoughts about your health, and you'll get discouraged and not follow through.

When those waves of uncertainty, doubt, and discouragement flood your mind, think like this: "Well, things are going a little slow; but, halleluiah, I'm making some progress. I'm confident I'm on the right path that will lead to better health and wellness. I had a rough day today, choosing the wrong foods and beverages, or skipping my workout. But I'm determined to make the very next choice a healthier one and keep on keeping on. I can see how I fell into that trap and made a mistake, and now have the ammunition to not have to make it again. Each day is a new day to live the healthy life I deserve".

Old habits and negativity must die. Be patient with yourself! Use the following mindful exercise to visualize anytime you can't seem to get past pitfalls or temptations.

Mindful Exercise: Visualization

Being a lifelong competitor and working with many different athletes as a sports dietitian, I have had the unique privilege to witness and learn about techniques elite and pro-athletes use to stay focused and overcome immense pressure to succeed.

Every sport on the planet uses visualization of some kind in the locker-room long before they ever step foot on the competition stage.

Let's use professional football and the Super Bowl as an example. Super Bowl Sunday sets the stage for the biggest game in NFL tradition, as two teams face off head to head. Millions of fans will gather together chowing down on chicken wings, assorted dips, and a variety of bubbling beverages.

Together they will sit in anticipation for the best commercials and an entertaining halftime show. Of course, all eyes will be awaiting legendary passes, fumbles, and points scored. And while viewers will go into the festivities unaware of how the game will unfold, the players and coaching staff have already exhausted countless hours rehearsing, drilling and visualizing potential winning plays.

Visualization has long been a part of professional and elite sports. It is the practice of mentally simulating competition from start to finish. Olympians have long known that taking time to imagine the perfect race, routine, or play, the better their chances of executing perfection under intense pressure. Coaches of all sports draw pictures, diagrams, and routes to show each individual player how to execute actions to achieve success. Over and over again, athletes physically and mentally visualize themselves executing the right moves and the right time. What looks like a lucky pass, catch, or kick has already been done countless times before, conceptually.

For those who are trying to eat healthier or move more, everyday life is a test of willpower to stay the course, and manage temptations without fumbling. Everyone can tackle the pressure to overindulge at get-togethers, caving into buying the same unhealthy foods, or not setting the alarm clock early enough to hit the gym by visualizing a healthy touchdown!

Go into each day or specific situation already envisioning you punting high-calorie foods, scoring extra points by drinking water, and sidelining mindless snacking by sticking to a one plate rule at dinner or parties.

Holiday season can be the worst or any celebration with food involved. Show up to the party well hydrated, without having skipped meals, and be ready to rumble with your friends, not the buffet.

Envisioning how you will intermingle, eat, and approach your greatest temptations may sound silly, but it works. This tool can help you reprogram your subconscious mind for dietary success, like a computer. If you truly struggle in one specific area then do this regularly, you will gradually notice a shift in your confidence levels and be able to handle any food choice more responsibly.

No one can truly pick the winner of Super Bowl Sunday or life beforehand, but you can bet that every player that takes the field knows the benefits of visualization for optimal outcomes. Overcome the nervousness and intimation of any wellness situation by taking a timeout and seeing yourself in action choosing healthy every time.

Chapter 6

Nix False Associations

*"There are some things one remembers even
though they may never have happened."*
— *Harold Pinter, Old Times*

The process of goal-setting begins with the question:
"What do I want?" We started this conversation in an
earlier chapter by completing a vision outcome from start
to finish. On the surface, it appears this should be an easy
question to answer. On the contrary, we may intellectually
know what we want, but with foods we are often driven by
how it makes us feel.

Whenever you try a new food, eat at a restaurant, or
engage in any kind of physical activity like running, a gym
class, or yoga, you either like the experience or you don't.
The way a food, certain menu item, or exercise makes you
feel in the moment, regardless if it is good or bad, becomes
a memory that stands as point of reference for you. You
measure subsequent food experiences against that
memory.

Everyone comes into the world with zero food
memory. In the beginning those memories are shaped by
your caregivers. They decide what your early memories
will be. In most instances that first memory will be of
mother's milk—or an animal substitute. Then maybe you
will progress to oatmeal or crème wheat. As you go
through childhood, you become more selective. You try

101

new things approved by your caregivers.

Often it is the forbidden fruit that you find most appetizing—hot dogs, French fries, sugar cubes, candy bars, etc.

All of this figures into your choices as an adult. As an adult, when you try new food items or restaurants, you make decisions based on your memoires of what you find tasteful or distasteful.

At some point you choose to try a new food, check out the latest restaurant and attempt the trendiest workout, all based upon how you expected (or hoped) the experience would make you feel. Most folks would not willingly subject themselves to anything guaranteed to be distasteful or painful.

The trouble comes when we intellectually want to make different choices than we have in the past, but find it almost impossible to override our old memories.

An extreme example of how past memories with food or beverage can alter your decision making for a very long time or indefinitely would be in the case of food poisoning. My dad is a grill king and one of his specialties used to be smoked ribs; they'd literally fall off the bone.

Like many Southern homes, we cook big on Sunday and eat leftovers throughout the week. No shame in that, but this particular time I had the unfortunate encounter with an illness after reheating and eating a few ribs for dinner.

If you have ever experienced food poisoning on any level then you have uttered the words, "I'm surely going to die!" Truth be told I am not 100 percent positive the ribs made me sick; it could have been something I ate three days before that finally took hold and made me ill. It could have been one of the side items I ate along with the ribs, or it could have easily been a stomach bug floating around at the time.

But, my perspective was that the ribs where the last to go down and the first to come up. The thought of the experience, lying on the bathroom floor wishing it would all just end still makes me nauseated. It was literally years before I could stomach another rib and to this day, it is not a favorite due to that one remembered experience.

In another instance, My husband became victim to a terrible case of food poisoning due to a meatball sub. I've never seen a grown man more sick than he became and neither of us have gone near a meatball sub or most meatballs ever since.

One encounter with food poisoning will influence your future behavior for a very long time. Sometimes the identified culprit is not really the source of the sudden onset of extreme illness.

A plate of ribs may be served with several side items and the ribs get the blame when it may have actually been the potato salad served along with the ribs. In fact, the illness could have been a stomach bug that can arrive unexpectedly and with great intensity. However, the experience taints innocent foods.

Same holds true past the plate and into the world of physical activity. Perhaps you make a commitment to exercise and you sign up for a boot camp although you haven't been active in several years. Your intention may be great and you are feeling all in.

On the first day you are pushed far beyond your limit, your blood sugar drops and you faint. Those memories become very powerful. Even if someone you know got injured doing a workout, whether it was their fault due to poor technique or overuse, you're less likely to push past fear and give it a go yourself.

Or, if your friend's older child got hurt playing a certain sport you will be more cautious of allowing yours to partake in a perceived dangerous activity later in life.

If you don't think you are so easily influenced by the memories of other people, then I encourage you to have lunch with a few toddlers and just observe what happens.

If one at the table takes a bite of a fruit or vegetable and enjoys it then the rest are more likely to follow suit. If one takes a nibble and spits it out the rest are sure to assume it's nasty, too. No convincing of how delicious it could be will work unless you can get just one to take your side and agree.

Daniel Kahneman, a Nobel Prize winning psychologist, and his team showed that the pleasurable quality of our remembered experiences is based on how the experience made us feel at its peak (best or worst), and how it made it us feel at the end. It is known as the Kahneman's "peak-end" rule and it is how the brain summarizes and categorizes experiences for future use in making decisions in similar situations.

When it comes to ordering in a restaurant many people fit perfectly into Kahneman's "peak-end" rule and rarely ever order something different off a menu.

If there is a Greek salad on the menu, I'm going to order it because I know, based on countless other tries, that it tastes good and meets my nutritional standards. There is nothing scientific about that choice. It may even be incorrect.

Therefore, while this can work in your favor, it can also backfire when you want to make positive shifts and feel like a failure when you make unhealthy decisions on autopilot. Imagine you are trying to eat healthier overall and made plans to dine out at your favorite Italian restaurant. For years you have ordered and enjoyed their creamy chicken Alfredo and homemade bread sticks. This time you had every intention to walk in and order a delicious salad and forgo the bread.

The moment you walk into the restaurant, all your senses are hit with "peak-end" experiences of pleasure. Memories of the laughs shared over dinner, the smell of the fresh bread, and sure enough someone is sitting at a table whirling their fork around a creamy pill of pasta. The waiter walks up and before you can stop yourself you have ordered chicken Alfredo and feel like what's the use in even trying to dine-out healthy. You'll start tomorrow.

When things like this happen, it is important to remember our previous exercises with meditation and visualization. Negative food memories can be overridden with the techniques we already have placed on the table.

* * *

Anyone not in the habit of getting up before work to

get in a jog or an exercise class understands this phenom-ena, too. The alarm goes off and without much resistance you push the snooze and roll right back over because everything in your body is screaming that sleep is more pleasurable than hitting the pavement.

No one can really blame you for sleeping in. You have no memory or experience that sweating before work would actually give you more energy than snoozing another half-hour.

Your past conditioning reinforced the feelings those familiar foods and habits provided. You've learned to continue to do what "feels good" based on experience.

What if I told you that many of our life's choices are derived from either trying to avoid pain or gain pleasure? You'd exclaim this is an over-simplification to your over-complicated life, but it's true.

Tony Robbins, a self-help trainer who bills himself as a "life coach," introduced me to the pain-pleasure principal in his book, *Awaken the Giant Within*, and it forever changed my understanding of human behavior.

His concept is simple. Every morning we wake up and move through the day making choices that will ultimately spare us pain or provide us pleasure. This is just another way to explain the psychological principle of gain and avoidance.

Gain and avoidance help determine where you live, what college you attend, who you marry, what shoes you put on today, or whether you order fries or salad at lunch. It guides whether you choose to be a marathoner or a couch potato, sky diver or stay planted on the ground.

This engrained principal is also what keeps many of you from taking the first step to make a committed decision with a purpose to attempt a new level of health and wellbeing.

In his book, Tony uses the example of procrastination to drive home the understanding of the gain-avoidance principal. We have all experienced procrastination at some point in time in life. Some people live in a state of procrastination and it is just how they function. But what ultimately is procrastination?

Procrastination is when you feel that the pain of doing something doesn't outweigh the pleasure of putting it off. Examples include: studying for an exam, compiling your taxes, expense reports for work, laundry, or a million other possible scenarios.

But, nature finally runs her course and there is a shift in your feelings toward the situation. Eventually the pain or consequences of not studying, filing taxes, submitting an expense, or washing clothes outweighs the pleasure of continuing to put it off.

Missing the deadline could cause you to fail, pay penalties, not get paid, none of which are pleasurable so you buckle down and get it done. You delayed action until it was no longer in your best interest or felt good to not evoke action. However, your health and wellness is arguably more important and valuable than a basket of dirty clothes.

Nothing like having a heart attack, hearing you have cancer, or may lose a limb to diabetes to make not changing your diet and lifestyle more painful than giving it a honest try.

Sadly, for some people, even after a heart attack, cancer diagnosis, diabetes, or high blood pressure still doesn't warrant enough pain to make a change for long-term pleasure.

Let this be your moment to become certain continuing your current lifestyle will bring unbearable, unnecessary pain in the future. Linking pain to the past, present and future will create a threshold that catapults you into finally taking action.

Unfortunately, most of us don't like to travel far from our memory bank and the present moment's neediness for pleasure. The problem is we think in terms of pain or pleasure in the short term instead of the long term and this influences our food, beverage, and exercise choices. A short minded mindset is what keeps you ordering French fries, desserts, and going back for seconds because it felt good last week and will surely feel good now. No thought of the future consequence.

Most of life's greatest gains often come from muscling through the short term pain to get to the long term pleasure of true good health. This could be a potentially life changing moment for you if you are willing to internalize that it isn't actual pain that always drives your decision making, but your perceived fear that something will lead to pain, displeasure, discomfort, distaste, or failure.

Same goes for pleasure. What drives us is the belief that some choice will bring enjoyment, comfort, taste, or safety. We are betting our choices on the feelings they will evoke. In other words, humans are not driven by reality but by our perceptions of reality and what we desire to feel or not feel.

If you have failed to take consistent action toward getting fit or healthy then be assured it is for one reason—at some point you began to associate more pain to getting healthy than not even trying.

Therefore, there is only one way you will ever make a lifelong change in your dietary habits or physical activity routine: without a doubt you have to associate sheer pleasure to all aspects of total wellness. Otherwise you will continue to make short term changes on fad-styled plans and never see the results of a long term commitment.

This is precisely why I loathe fad diets, weight loss challenges, or food fast of any kind. You mustard up the discipline to put yourself through diet torture, counting down days to freedom.

Sure you see measureable success in the short term, but you were so busy surviving you had no energy left to focus on learning the balanced way of doing things over the long term. Having tunnel vision to eliminate all sugar, only eat grapefruits, or drinking two shakes a day doesn't teach one thing about eating. It only better instills how to diet.

I am truly saddened to see someone force feeding themselves salads or vegetables or tossing the bun off their burger while gazing over at someone else eating a sandwich or pasta with shear envy in their eyes. Nothing makes a lunch date more awkward than a friend on a freaky diet who stares at you while you enjoy a sensible meal.

Until you change your opinion about the wholesome whole foods that are the only guaranteed way to sustain wellbeing or weight loss, you'll always feel punished and deprived and fall of the wagon into a pile of doughnuts and pizza slices.

I'll admit it is very hard for me to comprehend how someone can view eating life sustaining foods as torture or punishment. My pain-pleasure principal is conditioned to appreciate the health and nourishment that comes from plant based foods and sustainably raised animals. I am grateful for the opportunity to sit down to a meal that offers life, not death.

Fruits, vegetables, salads, whole grains, dairy, seafood, nuts and seeds, lean meats and water should all be viewed as the utmost privilege to eat and never as a penalty. Although food marketers and advertisements work hard to confuse you into believing your missing out if you don't indulge in fat, salt and sugar daily.

Will power is not enough to keep you ordering broccoli over French fries for a decade or more. You must learn to link healthy choices to true pleasure. Broccoli and foods that follow suit offer you years to spend with family, friends, doing the activities you enjoy, and the energy to get the 'greater purpose' out of this lifetime.

Pain should be linked to fries and other unhealthy foods and be seen as the grand-reaper slowing sucking away the one thing everyone wants more of, time. It is very difficult to see the long-term benefits of a healthy lifestyle. Reinforcement increases the likelihood of repeating or increasing a behavior. But reinforcement must occur soon after the desired behavior.

Trying to rely only on how much better your health will be in 20 years of healthy living usually isn't a strong enough reinforcer. You must develop reinforcement that is immediate. Maybe a self-congratulation note, marks on your vision chart or even a sliver of dark chocolate might be enough to keep you moving forward.

As we get older and take notice of our peers at family and high school reunions you may experience an epiphany (a sudden and striking reality) of the health of those who have maintained a healthy lifestyle and those who have not. Until you reverse the links in your brain you will never enjoy an anxiety free decision-making process while ordering off a menu or shopping for groceries.

Understand that there is a time and place for those unhealthy foods to fit into a well-balanced diet. I want you to understand that you have created false associations to foods that offer you zero long term benefits. While you may enjoy them in the moment they are causing you more pain and self-grief in the long-run.

For the love of good health: Stop holding on so tightly to the very things that are slowly killing you from the inside out.

This phenomenon of the pain-pleasure principal is rooted in real science. And while you may be feeling sort of down on yourself because of your false associations, the good news is we can all learn to condition our minds and emotions to link pain or pleasure to whatever we choose.

That is a simple secret to every person who has lost

weight and kept it off, quit smoking and never started back, and picked up running and competes in marathons into their senior years. They finally feel in love with a balanced and healthy lifestyle and remember the pain associated with old habits.

By changing our relationship to the behaviors that will garnish the results we desire we can start making healthier choices. This is my personal truth—to come to grips that my desire was to be strong. But I was addicted to thin. This is a mental battle that many physically active females (and women in general) face before every workout.

Pumped and prepared for a heart pounding, stress relieving hour, sweating away the cares of the world; I would suddenly be taken over by the fear of 20-inch biceps or thunderous thighs like the males in the weight room.

My inner athlete screamed to push harder, run faster, and lift more; but I had linked pleasure and self-value to thinness. The pain of not being the skinniest version of me outweighed the possible pleasure allowing my body to grow strong. So, I would dial back, re-rack the heavier weight and just continue to daydream about what strong would be like.

Learning this pain-pleasure principal and unlocking the false associations I had with being skinny by the world's standards allowed me to finally pursue my strong dreams. Not every woman wants to toss weights around, nor should they. But every woman can achieve strength With effort and stand strong in the body they were born into.

You will never regret pushing past your current threshold and linking pleasure to reaching your strongest potential in any area of life.

Another common area of false associations is found in the clean plate club. Are you a member? Dangerous grounds for anyone who struggles with their relationship with food. On the other hand, if you grew up in a food insecure home but found yourself in better living circumstances later in life, you may be hardwired to not let a morsel go to waste. Clean plate club members have linked pain to walking away with food left on a plate and pleasure to not being wasteful.

By now you can tell this is a very disempowering association with severe consequences. One must first become aware of this linkage and then proceed with reconditioning the mind to link pleasure to pushing the plate away with food left. Congratulate yourself, smile and acknowledge the good feelings of stopping when full.

The potential false associations in the realm of health and wellness are limitless and unique to each individual. A few of the strongest to break are the pleasurable false associations linked to the unhealthy foods.

Not only do you need to work to redirect the pain associated with vegetables to pleasure, but also the strong pleasure attached to sodas, cookies, chips, and all things fried.

I challenge you to see that what is truly the pleasure in those moments is the connection, communion with others, and time spent with those laughing, sharing, and being present.

Since what is truly pleasurable can't really be seen or measured our brains find any means to link the positive, pleasurable emotion too and it lands on the food or beverage that is within reach.

Easy to do since those items in themselves are pleasurable, but it's the moments not the menu item that makes our heart sing.

Learning your false associations or uncovering those hardcore remembered memories is the key to unlock the results you have never been able to achieve before. However, as the saying goes, "simple isn't easy." It takes a lot of self-awareness, authentic effort and committed choices to stay the course to create new memories.

Stick with it. The running theme here is you will create new associations little by little.

Mindful Exercise:
Reward to Rewire Your Associations

Did you know it is possible to teach a pig to push a shopping cart? Furthermore, you don't even have to demonstrate how it's done. I'm not crazy; researchers actually trained a hungry pig to push a cart. Using positive reinforcement, researchers provided treats to the pig every time he made progress with the cart. With a little patience the swine was able to strut around the room, pushing a cart like a seasoned shopper.

The concept comes from the psychological school

known as behaviorism and its most basic hypothesis: anyone will repeat behaviors that are positively reinforced with a prize or pleasure, and avoid behaviors that are negatively reinforced with punishment or pain. Although it isn't a fool-proof plan, we can all use it to increase the chances of adopting healthier behaviors.

Starting to embark on a weight loss or better health journey can be draining on your psychological and physical energy. Any big life change brings some fear, perceived failures, and disappointments.

Of course the success of losing weight, coming off medications, or reaching fitness milestones is exhilarating, but often those rewards don't come fast enough to combat the negative emotions first. That is why I highly encourage positively reinforcing healthy behaviors daily.

For instance, maybe you have a big-audacious-goal to lose a considerable amount of weight or complete your first marathon, neither of which could be conquered within a day's effort. You wake up on day one of your new journey faced with your first temptation: co-worker's birthday cake.

You know it isn't your birthday, but your reasoning probably goes like this: "On one hand there's my health. On the other hand, there is cake! Health, cake: cake, health. Health..... Just a little piece won't hurt."

We tend to think like the pig in the shopping cart experiment over the short term. Even though we have long-term goals we truly desire to achieve, our behavior is powerfully shaped by the lure of immediate rewards.

When the end seems so far out of sight we are more

apt to pursue the short-term pleasures even when it may not lead you toward your long-term objective.

Once you understand how false associations are driving your food and behavior choices you can feel downright hopeless to override those with simple will power. Since many of the false associations with food come from the pleasurable experience it seems to offer us it is smart to fight fire with fire and link positive associations with the behaviors you want to enjoy.

If you think I'm asking you to bribe yourself to eat healthier, drink water, and go for a walk, you're absolutely correct! In the beginning, doing the unpleasant but necessary tasks of ordering unsweetened beverages over soda, or vegetables versus fries isn't always joyful. Therefore, I'm offering you a way to get an immediate high-five feeling since you won't drop five pounds with every glass of water or bite of broccoli.

These pre-planned rewards will provide enough consistent short-term gratification to build the trust and enjoyment to help you stick with the long-term plan and reap the real results of better health. Don't make this complicated or pricey.

A productive positive reward is anything that sparks a smile. It could as simple as eating a healthy dinner off your favorite china that never gets used. Or decorate a water bottle that speaks to your unique personality.

Keep attractive flowers on the dinner table or display fruit in a fancy bowl. Reserve a sensible square of dark chocolate for a delicious treat to end a healthy, balanced and well portioned dinner. You could even leave your reward to the end of the day with a bubble bath or relaxing lotions.

If you like public accountability and affirmation post or share your meals on line and let your network of friends and your family know that you are trying to eat healthier and need their support. That certainly isn't an ideal reward for everyone, if the world wide web of opinions scares you (it does me) then just find a small support system and hold each other accountable and the reward of showing off your good choices will fuel the flame to keep on keeping on. You could get very creative with your family, co-workers, or faith-based community and create reward coupons. Once you have gathered enough you cash them in for a new pair of walking shoes, a cook book, or 5-K program. Or literally put a dollar or five (dependent on your budget and target purchase) into a mason jar every day or week you hit your fitness goals, drink plenty of water, or made visible improvements in your food journal. Once you've wracked enough cash then splurge on whatever your heart desires that isn't food.

The bottom line is to give a mindful thought every day to give yourself rewards: one for every healthy choice you make and at least one just because you're doing your best.

Chapter 7

Build Better Beliefs

"A belief is not merely an idea that the mind possess. It is an idea that possesses the mind."
—Robert Oxton Bolton

The strong link between our thoughts and the quality of our health has been the major theme of this book. Our inner dialogue is the source of much of our encouragement. Sadly, it is also the source of much of our discouragement.

All of us have had experiences that shape our thoughts. Some experiences offer hope and excitement about life and new adventures and then other experiences burn deep scares into our thoughts and create barriers and roadblocks to future experiences.

Some parents, family, teachers and friends give powerful messages that often guide youngsters to very rule- bound lives. They are taught that rules/laws are there to provide limits and expectations.

They are to be followed and never challenged. And, if you follow the rules you will be accepted, loved and protected. It can set some individuals up to seek perfection at a great personal cost. It is a philosophy of negativism, bombarding the person with "you should, you ought to, you must, don't, stop, etc. "

There is nothing wrong with being a law-abiding

citizen; it's our civic responsibility. Families tend to set up their own structure of family laws and expectations, and not all are healthy or based on promoting good mental health. And many are not designed to give young people the opportunity to learn from mistakes in order to develop their own moral compass.

Case History

Some of the best and worst advice Erin ever received was from her dad. He was a true man of integrity, and desired for his kids to do right and always choose the higher road. With the best intentions he gave Erin a little piece of advice when he gave her her first set of car keys at the age of sixteen. His gift was punctuated with a warning: "I will not tolerate a speeding ticket in this house. It's very easy not to get one, just don't speed."

Some adults lay the law down, by proclaiming what will and will not be tolerated. This tactic can without trying either intimidate the child into compliance or challenges the strong willed child to choose non-compliance. Then in some communities the fear of God and disobedience to him will result in eternal punishment.

These approaches are usually well intended and may be a result of their own upbringing or a genuine effort to protect those they love. It may be the only model they know. However, this model is based on fear and submission rooted in a negative tone.

Hopefully this book will help you evaluate your personal path that guides your life and decision-making, even beyond healthy living. If you operate solely from a negative or punitive base you will be constantly condemning and berating yourself. Negative thoughts begets disappointment and shame; whereas, positive thoughts beget courage, happiness and encouragement.

The father's advice was meant to keep his daughter safe and out of harm's way. Like I said, very well intended to keep her safe and out of harm's way. It was not the only time Erin's parents instilled in her that rules were in place for a reason and should always be followed.

Growing up in the Christian faith, it was reinforced that sinners (rule breakers) got punished by going to Hell and God isn't pleased with those who disobey the Ten Commandments.

It didn't take long for Erin's young mind to translate all the well-intended guidance to a belief that if she looked perfect, lived perfectly, and did everything perfectly, she would forever be protected from shame and failure. It doesn't take a psychiatrist to point out this is a destructive mindset that never leads to a happy ending. And it didn't. Erin ended up battling perfection for most of her life.

Anytime she found herself engaging in "bad conduct" whether that was partying in college, slipping a cussword, or eating a cupcake, her inner heckler would swoop in for the emotional beating. The voice had so much merit because her greatest fear was disappointing God, her parents, professors, bosses, or comrades.

Perhaps your inner troublemaker isn't the perfection police, but I bet you have your own heckler leaving in your head and it says the same negative, demeaning things to you day-in-day-out. The worst part about these inner comments is they develop into the belief system you live by and set you up for self-doubt, fear, and disappointment.

There are different methods a therapist might use to help you learn to stay on the positive thinking path. From wearing a rubber band on your wrist and snapping it when you recognize yourself turning down that path to one that is often used called setting a mental trap. With the mental trap it can be fun to give a name to the negative monster, maybe call it Freddy.

When your Freddy emerges with mean things to say that are setting you up to self-sabotage, condemn, frighten, or just hate on you, immediately call it out. A loud internal, "Shut up Freddy," can do the trick. And then immediately change what is being said, you ultimately control your thoughts.

Once you have the awareness to notice it, you now have choices. After the heckler has spoken, change your tonality to a confident comforter and reply with something really pleasant or funny. Respond to its tone that communicates, "You can't. You will never succeed" to more of a protective self roaring back, "Yes I can. Yes I will. Go away. You're not welcomed here." Notice how the changing of your tone to yourself makes you feel about yourself and about what you are attempting to do.

First getting acquainted with your thoughts, both internal Freddy and your positive self, evolves into your subconscious belief system. We all have a set of core principles that shape and determine every decision we have ever made and will make. What and how we believe consequently has a huge impact on what we do and whether we succeed or self-sabotage or even get out of the gate to try. So your thoughts determine your beliefs or feelings, which dictates your behavior. That is why concentrating solely on efforts to change behaviors such as eating, exercise or general lifestyle often fails until the preliminary work is done to identify and modify the root of the behaviors.

A simple analogy might be to consider our behaviors as the flowers on a tree. To truly change the flower you must go below the flowing bud. You can add nutrients to the soil or make sure it gets more sunshine or water. Just wanting and wishing for bigger and more colorful blooms doesn't make it happen no matter how much you rely on your wishes, without specific actions.

Other strong influences on developing and maintaining health and wellness come from those around you. Children, adolescents and even adults watch those around them. We usually have at least one person who is a strong influence on our life: parent, sister, or teacher. They serve as a role model that we try to emulate.

As we associate with those around us, our thinking, feelings and behaviors are affected and our belief system is developed. Some of us have a belief system that is rigid with no room for opposing ideas or beliefs; while many of us are open to new ideas and are more tolerant of differences among us.

Most people live by a belief system that they accept without much thought. Some of us go with the flow and never challenge why we believe the way we do but others may challenge traditional or cultural beliefs.

Life Lesson:
The only beliefs you should ever challenge are your own

What are beliefs? The simple answer is a belief is an assumed truth. A wider definition is that beliefs are our interpretations of the truth based on examination of evidence.

Every belief could be represented as a tabletop. For a tabletop to stand firm it needs legs, which represents the personal and compelling evidence your unique individual life has provided you.

Let's exam the belief, "I can't lose weight or keep it off." To support this belief you would tell me you've lost weight many times and it comes right back. You've tried every diet book on the market, but still crave cookies, chocolate, and slip back into old habits. Maybe everyone in your family carries extra weight.

Or, you just assume you're big boned. All life circumstance that becomes the legs that support the belief you can't lose weight or keep it off.

Everyone's thought patterns are comprised of two categories of beliefs: limiting or enabling. My favorite ways to classify them are as blocking or boosting beliefs. Limiting beliefs hold us back in life and enabling beliefs move us forward. I first became aware of the benefits of dividing beliefs into two categories from author and motivational speaker Tony Robbins, who used the terms "empowering" and "limiting" in explaining that beliefs can shape our behavior.

Limiting beliefs block infinite possibilities, boosting beliefs lead to growth, success and happiness. Enabling beliefs are not foolish beliefs. It is foolish to believe you could fly; it is boosting to believe you could learn to safely sky dive.

So, if enabling beliefs boost us into success and happiness, why don't we all just think those? Blocking beliefs are often built in safety nets to subconsciously keep us from doing anything too risky.

Boosting beliefs often lead us to taking risks, which naturally leads to the occasional perceived failure—man's mental nemesis.

Ironically, highly successful people are equipped to use more enabling beliefs to get through perceived failures, recover, learn, and carry on more prepared to make it the next time.

You know there is an absolute necessity to eating healthy, getting in physical activity, scheduling yearly medical exams, and drinking your water, but you resist it. It can be really useful to simply ask yourself, "What's stopping me?" or "Who said I can't?" or "Who believes I shouldn't?" or "Why am I resistant?"

And then listen for an answer.

You might be surprised to discover how much of your life is still being ruled by the insecure, unpredictable wisdom of a sixteen-year-old or your overprotective parent.

Case History

During Hannah's pregnancy she started enjoying a piece of dark chocolate after every meal. Since she needed a few extra calories daily it wasn't that big of deal. Post-delivery and trying to get the baby weight off she realized she still craved chocolate whether she needed it or not.

After paying attention for a while, she realized that after she finished a meal her mouth would literally start to salivate in anticipation of the chocolate. She would receive the same sense of relief and enjoyment from that piece of chocolate as one would describe from an after meal cigarette.

The sequence of events, finishing a meal and anticipating the sweetness filtered through her mind, and the feeling of satisfaction triggered the compulsion to eat the chocolate. Without conscious awareness, it became almost an obsession with her keeping chocolate squares in her purse at all times. She believed she had to have it or she wouldn't be able to be satisfied.

There is nothing wrong with a piece of chocolate after a meal, but the problem was that she didn't have a choice about it. It was self-defeating that she couldn't give up a silly piece of chocolate and go without it.

Once she realized this belief "I have to have chocolate" was blocking her from overcoming other issues in her life. If you are a slave to one bad habit you'll be more likely to become enslaved to others, too. Hannah tackled it head on and became so empowered when she realized she didn't "need" the chocolate and could enjoy it on occasion just fine.

Other words or phrases to be on guard for are massive overgeneralizations. We get into the habit of using words like all, always, every, and never when it comes to describing our abilities, inabilities, or capabilities.

Listen for them when you're talking, especially when you are talking about your health and wellness struggle. Listen to other people, too.

Sometimes it is easier to spot it in them first, but know they aren't along in their blocking beliefs—you just may not be willing to hear yours, yet. These red-flag words are like the red-flags on the beach, they stop you.

When you catch yourself thinking of saying, "oh, I'll never lose the weight," or "Every time I try to exercise something comes up," it is useful to determine where the belief came from.

What past life circumstances are giving it legs and is there a smokescreen standing between your belief and reality? Do you really believe you could never lose weight? No matter what you ate or drank or how much you moved, you'd never ever be able to lose a single pound?

Keep in mind that if you accept that you will never lose weight or get moving more, you'll be right. It's like Henry Ford said: "Whether you think you can, or you think you can't- you're right."

Mindful Exercise:
Build A Better Belief System

Your beliefs are literally an embedded command within yourself. Your ability to take action or avoid action in any given situation is triggered by your beliefs.

Let's learn to build a better belief system that enables to you get where you want to be and doesn't block or hinder your efforts.

Without over-thinking or over-analyzing, jot down every blocking belief you have in the area of eating healthy, drinking water, getting enough rest, or being physically active. Get real honest with yourself. Here are a few ways limiting beliefs appear in your internal dialogue.

I cannot:

I am not:

I am someone who does not:

I don't:

I don't have the courage to:

People like me don't:

I will never be able to:

I just don't like:

I don't deserve:

I must not:

Why do we limit our beliefs? We form beliefs through our direct experiences. We act, something happens, and we draw quick conclusions. Sometimes this is helpful, most of the time it just very limiting. Touching fire once and drawing the conclusion fire is dangerous-helpful. Trying to give up sodas, cigarettes, or chips just once and then drawing a conclusion you just can't – limiting.

Labeling yourself as a person who does not or cannot do certain things is a great excuse for inaction.

After you do a personal review of limiting beliefs, then spend time converting them into enabling or boosting beliefs. You can also look for other boosting beliefs to adopt. Your internal dialogue should go something like this to help boost you forward.

This might work. So it's worth giving it a go.

I can get there. I just need to keep going.

I am able. If I work hard, I can:

I am determined to:

I am a person who:

I am willing to:

I am capable of:

I deserve:

I am worthy of:

I will:

I am going to:

To conclude, literally rip up, burn, or run over the list of blocking beliefs. Then, every day take time to work hard at rewiring your brain for boosting beliefs. Repeat the list of enabling statements each day until they become committed to memory and effortlessly appear when a blocking belief arises.

The boosting beliefs can become personal mantra to also help transform your personal communication discussed in Chapter 2. Jotting a few down on several index cards and leave them where you will see them in your most used places: bathroom sink, work station, car, as book marks, or make them the background on your computer or smart phone. They cannot be powerful if they are not meditated on regularly and ready to slip off your tongue and easy as your ABC's.

Beliefs lead to an attitude, which determines your actions, which dictate your results.

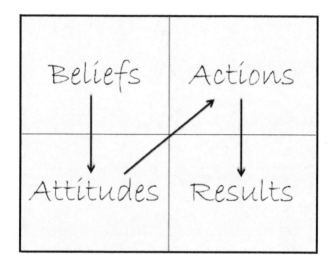

Chapter 8

Change Your Story

"Storytelling is the most powerful way to put ideas into the world today."
–Robert McAfee Brown

My dad introduced me to storytelling. He takes pride telling me an anecdote from his childhood or about some of the true characters within our family tree. But around every corner there is a story to be told.

Each person can recount their life's events, whether intriguing or not. It's their story to tell.

But your autobiography is a narrative that cannot be changed. Let's talk about the story you retell daily that nobody else hears, the memoir of your mind.

Remember, one of the healthiest things you can do is become aware of how you are talking to yourself. Let me continue to stress that you must think about what you are thinking about.

If you have implemented the mindful exercises of evaluating your inner communication, locating false associations, and discerning your blocking beliefs, then hopefully you are able to see a distinct pattern.

Our conversation with ourselves comes from our interpretation of our life. No one lives by the facts of life. We live according to the story we tell ourselves about the facts of our life.

Fact: You work full time, have children, and over

commit your spare time. **Story:** Life is chaos and finding time for physical activity is a joke.

Fact: Money is tight and there are bills to be paid. **Story:** Eating healthy is out of my budget.

Fact: You have tried every fad diet, quick fix, and magic pill and never been successful. **Story:** I am a failure with food so why bother trying?

Fact: You've never really tried addressing any of these mental obstacles before.

The good news is your conversation with yourself can change, starting today! The facts of your life may not change overnight, but your perception certainly can.

Now that you are aware of your inner monologue, try re-writing your own story. Since our thoughts create the world we see, it is a powerful tool to paint the picture we wish to live.

Instead of using your words to describe your current unhealthy situation day in and day out, use them to change your situation. This is where all the exercises come together to help you create a new story of your life. This entire chapter is designed to help you rewrite your health and wellness destiny.

Now take out that vision board and list of boosting beliefs you have been working on. You are already armed with all the tools and tactics to sit down and rewrite the ending to your life's story.

Take a few minutes and look over the vision board and empowering beliefs and begin to daydream about the type of person it would take to make it all jump off the paper and into reality.

Are you a rock climber who's learning to cook your favorite foods in a more healthful way? Or, a mom dedicated to limiting the sugar, fast foods, and fried fares for her family by replacing those with wholesome options.

Maybe you're a future marathoner with medals around your neck, strong legs attached to your feet, and an appreciation you have earned those splurge meals with your workouts.

Possibly you finally see yourself standing in the mirror, with a smile on face, and peace in your heart, because you finally appreciate and accept your imperfections and know you are doing your best, daily.

No matter what your goals and aspirations are you must start to see yourself as the hero of your life. When I decided to sit down and write a story for my life I drew inspiration from American scholar Joseph Campbell's *The Hero's Journey*. What better place to grab ideas from than a timeless pattern of narrative that appears in classic dramas, myths, religious rituals, and tall tales.

The Hero's Journey describes the typical adventure of the archetype known as the Hero, the character who goes out and achieves great deeds. It is about time you start to see life as an adventure and you as the hero or heroine seizing each new day as an opportunity to conquer the world at your fingertips. No more mundane Monday to Friday and living for the weekend. Heroes use every day as an opportunity to thrive and excel.

According to Campbell, there are twelve stages to the classic Hero's Journey. His first stage is rooted in the ordinary world. Perhaps you desire to be healthy and physically fit, but the lures of old unhealthy patterns of behavior weigh on your shoulders.

Or the fears of letting go of a comfort level of living and stepping into the unknown of new foods, new schedules, and new risks. You move to the second stage when you respond to a call for adventure. It may not be to sail the Seven Seas. Instead, it could be the diagnosis of diabetes, cancer, or rising blood pressure.

Maybe it was the reality that you need to be healthy to see your grandkids someday, or an internal nudge that you aren't living up to your full potential and life has much more to offer if you cleaned up your diet and exercised more. Campbell's third stage is one he calls the refusal of the call. The hero feels the fear of the unknown and tries to turn away from the adventure.

We've all been here before. Maybe you have tried every fad diet on the market or have declared Monday as the turnaround point a thousand times with no lasting results. This could represent the unfortunate yo-yo cycle that has represented the last few years or decades of your life. You heard the call, you sort of accepted it, and then you refused.

Campbell's fourth stage is one he called "meeting with the mentor." The hero typically comes across a seasoned traveler of the world who gives them advice, tools, tactics, or training that will help on the journey.

Or the hero finds the guideline light within and a source of inner courage and wisdom. Let me just go head and beef up my ego and assume I am your guide light on this health and wellness journey. Let this book be the kick in the rear that finally resonates that you have all the tools within you to live an abundant and healthy life.

I won't go through all of Campbell's stages (you can read the book for that), but I challenge you to examine your life in the context of his vision of life being composed of one stage after another until completion.

Here is where you finally bring your entire vision board to life and harness the personal power you have created and pay it forward. Holding onto all the secrets that set you free from your mental bondage won't help anyone, including yourself. Sowing the seeds into other will only strengthen them within you. You will be the catalyst for someone else's healthy hero journey.

Visualizing how you wish your life to unfold and being wise enough to factor in the most common roadblocks will catapult you into success. Writing this vision and story down will better ensure you will withstand the highs and lows that come with any hero's quest to self-improvement.

The difference between a movie and real life is we are all constantly on the Hero's Journey until we part ways with this ordinary world. You may conquer health and wellness and then if you are open to it, life will show you a new path to start the process all over.

Don't ever stop adding chapters to your life story.

Your thoughts will determine the foods you choose, the beverages you drink, the exercise you engage in, and ultimately your future. The idea you are exempt from being able to achieve a balanced and healthy lifestyle is all in your mind. You can think yourself into an unhealthy mess or you can think yourself into a place of better health and victory.

Don't just write a killer story and then toss it in a draw somewhere. Keep this precious dictation of your future success out front and visible. Mind Over Fork is one of the hardest habits to achieve and keep under control. The meditation exercises laid out in the first chapters are tools to guard you against negative mindsets.

Good health or positive thinking doesn't just happen. Good health is within your reach, no matter where you are starting from, and I need you to hear yourself say that you believe it too.

Remember, you are actually "talking" to yourself all the time, even right now. So why not just make an effort to talk nicely to yourself every day, no matter how badly you think you screwed up.

At the dawn of each day, read and affirm your new story and boosting beliefs. Having your mind in the right state before the day begins is so important to your success. Your thoughts create the world you see. Change your story, change your life.

Chapter 9

Reflect to Progress

*"Life can only be understood backwards;
but it must be lived forwards."*
— Søren Kierkegaard

As we move into Part Two, it's the perfect time to remember why we started the Mind Over Fork to begin with. After implementing the mindful exercise over a period of time there will be some lessons learned that will better equip you to actually succeed at making real change with the information provided in Part Two.

Life's best teachers are our individual experiences, if you allow them to be. Reflection is thinking about and linking experiences, looking for commonalities, differences, and patterns. The goal is to identify precisely the behaviors you wish to address and become aware of how it appears in all its ugly forms in order to effectively problem solve.

True reflection goes deeper than, "I eat too many cookies," or "I have a false association to chocolate." It is seriously looking back, utilizing all the mindful exercises provided and uncovering what lies between you and your health goals. Why? Because, in the upcoming chapters, you'll never succeed at implementing my food solutions if you don't fully understand what has kept you from sticking with healthy eating.

Before diving into what seems like the "good stuff,"

reflect in such a manner that it challenges your beliefs, cultural practices, and social structures in order to assess their impact on your daily habits. Remove the rose colored lenses and face your reality to aid you in cultivating resolutions that will work. Imagine alternative ways of thinking, doing, and living in order to provide a fertile ground for change that will propel you forward with my food solutions.

If your reflections are still discouraging and you are guarded to fully commit to this process because of the fear of being disappointed, I want to remind you how worthy of good health you are and that it is obtainable.

If you suffer from self-doubt or poor self-image, if you abuse your body with unhealthy foods or unhealthy habits, even if you simply put yourself last on the list, under the family, work, or social groups, then you may not understand or respect your own value.

If you truly valued yourself you would not abuse your body. Everyone was put on this earth for a purpose, and no one can fulfill their highest potential by forfeiting their health.

You were born with the right to be healthy. You were born with the right to love yourself, to enjoy life and to reach your full potential. Don't resist making the changes you know are necessary.

Take heart, there is healing available to any and every one who seeks it. Somewhere along the way you may have forgotten your worth, buried it under a to-do list and the demands of a fast paced family. Today's typical schedule is one that clamors loud for our 24-hour attention.

Some of us ascribe to a tarnished value system by placing money, status and stuff ahead of mind, body, and spirit. I can't tell you how important it is to not only reform your diet, grocery list, and cooking style, but also your value system. To truly create a balanced and healthy lifestyle you must put your entire being (body, mind, will, emotions, and spirit) right at the top of your to-do list. Only can you maintain a level of healthy living and reach your full potential if you keep the entire package in focus.

Let me give you an example. The nature of my work requires me to travel and to be available to the public. The trick lies in learning how to balance making it happen and letting it happen.

The hardest word in the English language to say is no! It never fails that my schedule is packed when a great opportunity pops up and I say sure I can show up, do it, or fit it in. As soon as the words "sure thing" comes out of my mouth my heart races in anxiety of how it'll all get done.

Eating your vegetables, drinking water, and being physically active will not protect your immune system from imploding when you lack sleep, quiet time, or are stressed to the max. Like clockwork, when I over-schedule or over commit myself, I end up with strep throat, the flu, or some other train wreck of an illness. *It makes since that disease happens when we are living in "disease."*

Remember, if you don't take good care of your body, your mind, and your soul you will be less effective with your goals in life. Worry, anxiety, stress, can't be fixed with a good diet and exercise. When we are mentally exhausted or weak, nothing will work right. You and I are complicated beings and each of our needs require proper care and attention.

That's what this book is about. I wrote it because I am saddened at the number of people I see—at daycare when I drop off my kid, even in the gym and the general public—who are not taking full care of themselves. Countless people clearly feel terrible.

Just look at how people carry themselves and listen to what they say, "I'm sick and tired," "I'm stressed to the max," "I can't sleep" "I have no energy"

It should be instinct to take care of ourselves. Pet owners know that dogs, cats, and even chickens eat when they are hungry, stop when they are full, play during the day, stretch upon waking, and take frequent naps. You don't see your pooch rushing around and lying awake at night worried about whether he'll get a bone tomorrow or not. So why don't we do the same?

We know how to diet, but not how to eat. Years of bad fad-diets, misinformation, infomercials touting miracles in a bottle, and easy access to fast food and pre-packaged food have left Americans remarkably confused about what a wholesome diet is and how they should eat.

We are submerged behind the skinny smokescreen. As mentioned in Chapter One, we are inundated with unattainable ideals of beauty, but ironically nearly half of Americans are overweight or obese. I fear we are inwardly striving for model perfection, but outwardly we are slowly normalizing obesity as an acceptable standard of living.

We are divorced from movement. History proves humans were built to be a body in motion. Physical activity was an integral part of our daily existence. Fundamentally, humans would never have excelled without immense physical capabilities.

Obviously, you no longer need to be able to run naked while carrying a sharp object to catch dinner. But, now we've developed so much technology that we often live completely detached from any physical activity past brushing our teeth and walking to our car.

This book does not go into an exercise program because it is not within my scope of practice. This does not negate the importance of physical activity. If you are currently sedentary, I urge you to begin to work up to 10,000 steps five days a week for good health.

Many have become hooked on selfless. Self-sacrifice can be addictive. Admit it; it feels good to do for others and it can make us feel important, or a false sense of value. Sure, helping others is important and families need their momma, but many women get out of balance with placing their family and career needs well above their own. Their suffering becomes their virtue, and then it becomes a problem.

We have forgotten our own self-worth. All roads

lead home and it is imperative that you internalize your own importance. Taking care of yourself should be mandatory not a luxury. Your body is the only house you get to live in, taking care of it makes good sense. Let's get started with changing the way you feed it.

Using the 5 Food Solutions for Weight-loss Success
The Great Wall of China was not built in a day, and neither was Rome or good health. Personal health is an ongoing pursuit. But like any big assignment, you begin with a solid strategy for success, and that's just what the second part of the book offers. The first half of the book tackled the mind and now we get to the fork.

I intend to help you begin, or jump-start a balanced and healthy lifestyle with five food solutions rooted in good science and my personal experience. It is time to stop repressing your desire to get fit, and address the patterns of behavior holding you back, to turn your "I wish" into "I will become healthy."

Eating healthy doesn't have to be daunting or mentally draining with counting calories, stressing over grams and ounces; is just not necessary.

In fact, that mindset is the very reason many don't even care to give healthy eating a try, it appears too complicated, and no fun! My philosophy is that you don't have to control every eating circumstance, but you can approach every situation in the most balanced way.

A strategy is a method or plan chosen to bring about a desired future, such as achievement of a goal or a solution to a problem. My five food solutions to healthy weight are so simple that you won't believe this is all it takes to be healthy and reach your goals for the long term.

This is not a diet. These are road signs or guiding lights pointing the way to the healthiest choices. The extent you want to follow these principals is up to you. That's the good part. Obviously, the more serious you are about implementing them, the better the results.

Each of the next five chapters discusses one key to building a lifestyle that nurtures balanced well-being without totally giving up life's delicious pleasures.

I'll explain what the strategy to the solution is and why it's so important to healthy weight success. And I'll arm you with practical, down-to-earth suggestions for incorporating them into your life. I don't expect you to do all five perfectly. Your task is to read each chapter, and be open-minded how to incorporate them into your daily life.

* * *

Each of the five solutions has a specific focus, but all of them overlap. You will get the most reward for your effort reinforcing them all at once.

The good news is that healthy behaviors encourage other healthy behaviors. If it does seem overwhelming then just pick one at a time and nail it down before moving on. There is no shame in taking it at your own pace.

But, you will probably find that as you go along, implementing each solution into your routine, it gets easier and easier. One day in the near future, you'll wake up and realize you have created an incredibly balanced and healthy life.

There's my pep-talk. Now continue your mindful exercises from Part One. They are your foundation to implementing what's to come to stick.

Stay hungry for healthy!

Part 2

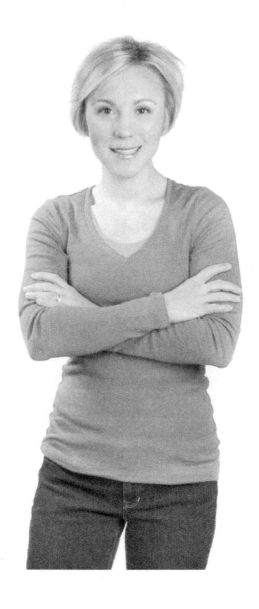

Chapter 10

Rethink Your Drink

"Thousands have lived without love, not one without water."—W. Auden

I know you have heard the spiel about drinking plenty of water a 1000 times, but for fun just listen to it one more time. Liquid calories are the number one cause of added sugars and un-necessary calories in most people's diets.

It is shocking how many calories some take in daily through the glass, bottle, tap, or straw. Rethinking what you drink is the easiest, most effective way to begin a health and wellness transformation.

The problem is liquid calories often go down so fast and smooth we tend to forget how much we drank throughout the day and the calories begin to really add up. Relatively speaking with an average caloric ranking, a person would rack up 1370 calories from just fluids if they simply consumed the following:

8 ounce orange juice: 110 calories
Medium Mocha: 400 calories
20 ounces regular soda: 280 calories
16 ounce fruit beverage: 230
16 ounce sweet tea: 200 calories
12 ounce beer: 150
= 1370 calories!

I doubt that you drink exactly that every day, but for most of us it is some combination. Do you love your fancy coffees, sodas, sweet tea, or adult beverages daily? Then take an honest account of what you are swigging and see how many extra calories are coming from the glass. You may be overwhelmed with the amount.

Take a big sigh of relief; this will be the easiest of all the five food solutions to straighten out if you are willing. I'm not asking you to nix it all, but I will firmly request you consider decreasing any beverage that holds a calorie to the following boundaries.

Drink half your body weight in water ounces every-day. Drink Unlimited: unsweetened tea, unsweetened green tea, or unsweetened coffee. Drink Sparingly: low-fat milk, no more than (2-3) 8 ounce glasses daily.

Limit to One: 100 percent fruit juice or fresh juiced to 6 ounces daily.

Limit to One: artificially sweetened or any other sweetened beverage.

Limit to One: Alcoholic beverage daily. Notice, I didn't say zero of anything!

Just a few tweaks in beverage choices can make a huge impact in the reduction of daily caloric intake and impact on overall health. Relatively speaking with an average caloric ranking, a person would lower their intake to 340 calories from switching fluids to the following:

8-ounce skim milk: 80 calories
Medium Non-fat latte: 160 calories

Diet Soda: 0 calories
Unsweetened tea: 0 calories
Water: 0 calories
Light beer: 100 calories

I am a warrior of water and take my coffee and teas unsweetened, but on occasion I will enjoy a diet soda and there are not many days that go by I don't enjoy a sensible glass of wine or local beer. I do not purchase soda or juice of any variety for the home, saves temptation and money.

And although decreasing your soda consumption from multiples to only one is a win in my book, I will still make the case for eventually eliminating sugar-sweetened beverages entirely. The Center for Disease Control and Prevention (CDC) published the "Sugar-Sweetened Beverage Consumption Among Adults in 2012—18 States In 18 states, more than 26 percent of adults consume sweetened-beverages such as regular soda and fruit drinks at least once daily. Sugary drinks are one of the primary sources of added sugars in U.S. diets and have been associated with a range of negative health outcomes including being overweight or obese.

As the CDC report noted, highly sweetened-beverage consumption is probably influenced by the food environment and beverage marketing. In fact, sugary drinks are frequently granted greater advertising space in grocery stores located in the Southern United States, where three of the five top states for sugar consumption are located.

150 calories and 44 grams sugar. A serving of sugar is a mere teaspoon at 15 calories and 5 grams of sugar, so that means there are 10 servings of added sugar and 100 percent of the calories come from sugar. For every can of soda you replace with a zero calorie beverage you could lose up to 10 pounds a year!

Still not convinced sugary beverages are worth nixing? Think about these opportunities to shed easy pounds and improve health. If you replaced a daily Double Gulp with water, you would reduce annual calorie intake by 209,875 calories or almost 60 pounds in a year. If you replaced a daily Big Gulp with water, you would reduce annual calorie intake by 125,925 calories or 36 pounds per year. If you replaced a daily large regular soda at any fast food chain, you would reduce annual calorie intake by 113,150 calories or 32 pounds per year. If you replace a daily medium (16 oz.) soda at any fast food chain, you reduce annual calorie intake by 54,750 calories or just over 15 pounds per year.

I hope you will truly consider saying goodbye to a daily dose of sugar-sweetened beverages. But before you just compromise to switching your carbonated habit to artificial sweeteners, I beg you to think twice. There is just no alternative to adequate water intake.

Artificial sweeteners are a hot topic of debate. Truthfully, there is not enough definitive scientific evidence, yet that makes me jump on either side of the fence. I will argue some artificial sweeteners are more natural, and potentially safer than others. Stevia is made from a plant and is my go-to choice. If you are currently a blue, yellow, or pink packet person, I encourage you to try to reduce and replace those with Stevia.

However, never should your artificially sweetened beverages outweigh the plain water or unsweetened beverages you drink. I understand that life deserves a little sweetness and using 1-2 packets or 1-2 teaspoons of Stevia a day offers an opportunity to enjoy a boost in flavor without added sugar or calories.

Artificial sweeteners used in a responsible manner can also offer those with Type 1 or Type 2 Diabetes the chance to enjoy life's sweetest treats without putting their delicate blood sugar in the danger zone.

Let me be clear: artificial sweeteners of any kind are NOT the answer to our sugar addiction. Both the American Heart Association and the American Diabetes Association have given only a cautious nod to their use. Dr. David Ludwig, an obesity and weight-loss specialist at Harvard-affiliated Boston Children's Hospital, is concerned that people who use artificial sweeteners may replace the lost calories through other sources, possibly offsetting weight loss or health benefits.

If you are holding on to your soda with death grips just let this sink in. Average 12 ounce cans of soda contain Non-nutritive sweeteners are far more potent than table sugar and high-fructose corn syrup," Dr. Ludwig explains. "A miniscule amount produces a sweet taste comparable to that of sugar, without comparable calories. Overstimulation of sugar receptors from frequent use of "these hyper-intense sweeteners may limit tolerance for more complex tastes."

The result of that, he explains, is that people who routinely use artificial sweeteners may start to find less intensely sweet foods, such as fruit, less appealing and un-sweet foods, such as vegetables, less palatable.

If you find yourself needing more than 1-2 packets of artificial sweeteners a day then you have a bigger issue with needing that "sweet taste" than you're willing to admit. You should take time to address that "need for a sweet taste" before searching out a healthier artificial sweetener.

Now before you give me the argument that regular sugar is better than anything artificial, just beware of how much sugar you are eating and drinking. Sugar, of all kinds (table, honey, agave etc.), causes an increased risk of over doing calories, being overweight, forming diabetes, and some cancers. The natural way doesn't always mean low-calorie and that certainly holds true for sugar.

Spotting sugars in foods and beverages is getting increasingly more difficult. A new term for sugar seems to pop up often in hopes to sneak it into products. To better educate you, here is a simple review of all the different types of sugars and their code names. This certainly holds true for drinks, which is the focus in this chapter, but it is also applicable to any food product. Get sugared educated.

Sugars These are carbohydrates and contain 4 calories per gram. They are found naturally in many foods including fruit, vegetables, and milk. Natural sugars offer the benefits of nutrients that cane or table sugar do not.

The most common are: Sucrose, Glucose, Dextrose, Fructose, Lactose, Maltose, Galactose and Trehalose.

Sugar Alcohols Like sugars these are carbohydrates and occur naturally, though in small amounts, in plants and cereals. They typically contain fewer calories per gram than sugar, because the body is unable to fully metabolize them. The downside of this is that they can cause cramps or bloating if taken in excess. The most common are: Sorbitol, Xylitol, Mannitol, Maltitol, Erythritol, Isomalt, Lactitol, Glycerol

Natural Caloric Sweeteners These are among the oldest known sweeteners and include honey and maple syrup. They contain sugar but also other nutritive qualities. They still need to be eaten in moderation as they can cause the same health consequences as any sugar in large quantities. They include: Honey, Maple Syrup, Coconut Palm Sugar and Sorghum Syrup.

Natural Zero Calorie Sweeteners These are not carbohydrates and contain little or no calories. It is only in recent years that interest has grown in these as a better alternative to artificial sweeteners. Like synthetic artificial sweeteners they can have an aftertaste and lead to bloating or gas if consumed in large amounts. They include: Luo Han Guo, Stevia, Thaumatin, Pentadin, Monellin, and Brazzein.

Modified Sugars These are typically sugars produced by converting starch using enzymes. They are often used in cooking or in processed foods. These should be consumed in the least amounts possible. A few are: High Fructose Corn Syrup, Refiners Syrup, Caramel, Inverted

Sugar, and Golden Syrup.

Artificial Sweeteners There are many types on the market and some appear to be safer than others. They have been in use in America and Europe for over 120 years. The most common are: Aspartame, Sucralose, Saccharin, Neotame, Acesulfame K, and Cyclamate.

While I heavily advocate for you to reduce and remove your liquid sugar calories, some sugars come from natural sources and contain other beneficial nutrients. Fructose found in 100 percent fruit juice with no sugar added or fresh squeezed juice contain pulp with fiber and wholesomeness. Fruit juice of any kind is still high in sugar and should be enjoyed in moderation, 6 ounces daily. Feel free to just eat the whole fruit for even more of a nutrition punch without as much sugar found in the juice.

My other go-to nutritious beverage is real cow's dairy milk. Research has long shown that dairy's nutrients are vital to the development of bones and reduce the risk for developing rickets and osteoporosis. A simple cup of low fat milk provides 30 percent of the daily value of calcium, a mineral that helps build and maintain strong bones and teeth. It's not just calcium that makes milk bone-friendly, dairy products contain other bone building nutrients including vitamins D, phosphorus, potassium, and protein.

Vitamin D not only helps our bodies absorb calcium, but also may boost immunity, reduce the risk for some cancers, and promote better blood pressure. Today all commercial fluid milk sold in the United States is fortified with vitamin D. At only 25 cents a serving, a single glass of milk delivers a package of nine essential nutrients important for good health.

While I am a champion for milk, let's not get carried away with the portion sizes. A serving of milk comes in the form of 8 ounce glass of milk, 6 ounce yogurt, or 1 ounce of cheese.

You only need 3 servings of a combination of these three to get the maximum benefits of its nutrients. Over eating or drinking any nutritious food or beverage still puts you at risk for gaining weight.

Are you or someone in your family one of the estimated 12 percent of the US population who has lactose intolerance? Lactose intolerance or sensitivity is the inability to digest the natural sugar lactose that's found primarily in dairy foods.

Some people do not have enough of the enzyme lactase, which breaks down the sugar within their digestive system. Lactose sensitivity symptoms include abdominal pain, diarrhea, gas and uncomfortable bloating. This food sensitivity can be difficult to diagnosis since symptoms can be attributed to a range of health issues.

The good news is that those with lactose intolerance can use lactose- free dairy products such as lactose-free milk, lactose-free ice cream, lactose-free yogurt, and lactose-free cottage cheese. Try foods with active or live cultures such as Greek yogurt with friendly bacteria to help digest lactose. Check out the dairy case. There are many more lactose-free products available than ever before.

You may still be trying to figure out how to limit alcohol to only one serving daily. I realize this can be a stinger for some readers who use it as a way to de-stress. I totally get it. Your glass or two of wine at night is your coping mechanism for a hard day.

The truth is the body doesn't know how to use alcohol so it ends being metabolized as a fat, regardless of the hard day you had. Since this is a total health and wellness journey, commit to finding other ways to de-stress that doesn't metabolize as an unnecessary fat.

According to the Dietary Guidelines for Americans, moderate alcohol consumption is defined as having up to 1 drink per day for women and up to 2 drinks per day for men. This definition refers to the amount consumed on any single day and is not intended as an average over several days.

The Dietary Guidelines also state that it is not recommended that anyone begin drinking or drink more frequently on the basis of potential health benefits because moderate alcohol intake also is associated with increased risk of breast cancer, violence, drowning, and injuries from falls and motor vehicle crashes.

According to the Center for Disease Control and prevent website: A standard drink is equal to 14.0 grams (0.6 ounces) of pure alcohol. Generally, this amount of pure alcohol is found in:

12-ounces of beer (5 percent alcohol content).
8-ounces of malt liquor (7 percent alcohol content).
5-ounces of wine (12 percent alcohol content).
1.5-ounces or a "shot" of 80-proof (40 percent alcohol content) distilled spirits or liquor (e.g., gin, rum,

vodka, whiskey).

Water: The First Nutrient

Water has been credited for being the reason for life on earth. All of earth's creatures, including humans, rely on water more than any other substance to maintain good health. We can live longer without food than water, and the efficient metabolizing and uptake of all other nutrients are impacted by the amount of water taken in.

The reason is simple: our bodies are about 60 percent water by weight, and most nutrients move around through our body in water. Our bloodstream is composed primarily of water, and so are all of our tissues and organ systems. Water is also the key to elimination of toxins from our body in the form of urine and perspiration (sweat). Even our ability to see, hear, think, sing in the shower, and laugh at life all depend on water.

Researchers at Loma Linda University looked at water consumption in a group of more than 20,000 men and women in their Adventist Health Study. In this study, they determined that adults drinking 5 or more glass of water each day were about 50 percent less likely to die from a heart attack. These researchers ranked increased plain water drinking as important to health as smoking cessation in terms of heart health! Just think if we all stopped smoking and drank our water how much healthier the world would be!

Appropriate water intake helps maintain proper blood pressure, improves mental performance, increases athletic performance, and helps regulate digestion. If someone suffers from occasional constipation or irritable bowel systems, the first place I start is their water intake. It takes a lot of water to soften and move food from start to finish.

There are three distinct categories for water benefits: lubricant, solvent, and thermostat.

Water is a lubricant. It keeps things flowing and moving. While it lubricates, water also protects our body parts from damage by surrounding them in a shock-absorbing fluid. This aspect of water is especially important in our joints, and also in our skin. The second aspect of water is its role as a solvent. Most nutrients dissolve in water. Especially our water soluble vitamins, the B vitamins—folate, thiamine, riboflavin, niacin, pantothenic acid, biotin, vitamin B6 and vitamin B12 -- and vitamin C. Also our electrolytes need water to work properly. The electrolyte minerals like potassium and sodium stay dissolved in water. The third aspect of water involves its role as a thermostat. When we are too hot, water lets us shed heat through sweating.

Water also helps us retain heat when we need to stay warm. It is amazing how many of our general aliments could be eliminated with adequate plain water intake.

So how much water should you be drinking daily? Hydration needs are individualized. It depends on weight, activity and temperature. The average person, not engaged in endurance sports, should consume half their body weight in ounces every day.

You may be shocked at the amount of water you need daily. However, the more body mass you have or the taller you are the more moving parts you have to lubricate, absorb shock from, and surface area to cool off or heat up.

Of course a petite person will require less than a taller person. So no excuse, do the math and drink up! Example: If you weigh 150lbs you should consume 75 ounces of water daily or 9-10 cups. Please, let's keep the health of our bodies and the planet in mind. Invest in a stainless steel or a BPA free water bottle to carry with you and forgo being a slave to bottled water. Finding a water bottle that expresses your own unique personality will also encourage you to drink water on the go.

If you aren't a water warrior already it may take some time to generate a true desire for plain water. Here are some amazing recipes to boost the flavor of your water without adding unnecessary sweeteners of any kind or calories.

The recipes read to be made in a large pitcher, but also try making them in individual mason jars that are portable and perfect for infusing flavors. Purchase a case of 8 to 12 large mouth mason jars; they will come in handy for many nutritious recipes.

Give each of these a try, feel free to tweak, and sip confidently knowing your beverage choice will help you stay hydrated, lose weight, reduce bloat, and reach your wellness goals.

Cucumber Lime Water
2 Liters water
1 cucumber, cleaned and thinly sliced
1 lemon, cleaned and thinly sliced
10-15 fresh mint leaves

Strawberry Grapefruit Water

2 liters water

3-5 strawberries, washed and sliced

1 medium cucumber, washed and sliced

1 small grapefruit, washed and sliced

Apple Pie Water

2 liters water

2-3 apples, washed, cored, and thinly sliced

2 cinnamon sticks

Blueberry Mint Water

2 liters water

1 pint blueberries, washed

7-10 mint leaves

1/2 lemon, washed and thinly sliced

For each recipe combine all the ingredients in a gallon pitcher and let sit in the fridge a minimum of 30 minutes, but best overnight. As mentioned, split the ingredients up into individual largemouth mason jars or water bottles for quick grab and go waters.

You can refill the water about 3 times before tossing the ingredients; just know the flavor will be slightly diluted each time. Get creative and come up with your own combination and fruits or vegetables to infuse in water and come share them online with everyone.

Chapter 11
Divide and Conquer

"Nothing is particularly hard if you divide it into small jobs."—Henry Ford

Tackling the first food solution of rethinking your drink leaves many visiting the bathroom more frequently. Others realize it is harder to commit to the adequate amount of daily water that is necessary for optimal health and that's okay, too. Never feel that perfection is the only road to success, in fact, perfectionist thinking gets in the way of positive progress. Keep making progress with your fluid choices and you'll see health and wellness results.

The second food solution, called "Divide and Conquer," dives into the meat and potatoes of your day and focuses on when you eat meals and snacks. I'm sure you've heard the advice to eat smaller meals throughout the day to maintain a healthy weight. But I want to give you the science behind why it's a good weight loss strategy.

I love the idea of being able to gain or maintain power by breaking things into more manageable pieces. And, that is exactly how your body and metabolism feel when you offer it a steadier stream of nutrients or food throughout the day, instead of large quantities at one time. Digesting, absorbing, and distributing of nutrients is made easier for the body when it's divided into small jobs.

After years of trying to educate groups of diverse people on how to think about eating, I've come to the conclusion that envisioning the body as a 24/7 factory gets the message across best. I want you to imagine your body's digestive and absorption systems as a factory that employs shift workers 24 hours a day, 7 days a week, and 365 days a year and relies on quality shift workers to get the job done.

If you have never witnessed a real life factory, it is still easy enough to image how it operates. Most factories operate everyday all year in concurrent shifts to produce a product such as cars, furniture, or packaged foods. Even logistic companies and the Post Office never stop moving. Shutting down even one day or a few hours may mean lost profits that can't really be made back in overtime due to production limits.

Even the most efficient factory has a max number of outputs per shift, due to equipment, space, and time for production to take place.

Every factory's management team knows the optimal number of employees to have at each shift to produce the max number of product based on equipment ability. Logistic companies know just the right number of drivers to have on hand to get the cargo distributed efficiently and cost effectively.

Neither more nor less employees on any given shift will improve production once max capacity has been hit. Your body's digestive system and metabolism works very much like a factory, except its output is to sustain real life and overall wellness.

Your factory (body) works whether you help it out or not, 24 hours a day, 365 days a year to keep you alive and as well as possible. The workers we employ on a daily bases to keep our body up and running in tip-top shape are nutrients found in the foods and beverages we consume. Macro- (carbohydrates, fats, and proteins) and micro- (vitamins and minerals) nutrients are the only workers we have access to, to get the job done.

How effective our factory is at maintaining good health depends on how efficient we are at employing the right type of nutrients at the right time of day.

In short, when we eat too little throughout the day, we are not providing the body with enough nutrients as our workforce to adequately get the refueling, renewing, or maintaining job done.

We will be fatigued, become sick, have a slow metabolism, and not reach any of our wellness goals. On the other hand, if we overload our body at any one given meal with too many nutrients or calories then the body will work with the number of nutrients it needed to run optimally during that shift, and unfortunately, the other nutrients not necessary at that time will be ushered to storage as fat cells.

I recommend people of all ages and activity levels maintain a steady intake of wholesome food and beverages every 3-4 hours. While this may sound like an awful lot, it isn't. For most people that translates to 3 full meals and 1-2 snacks, daily.

When we routinely stick to providing the body with nutrients about every 3-4 hours we will optimally digest and metabolize the nutrients for good health and wellness. No task will be left undone such as repairing; recovering, rebuilding, and no extra nutrients will be left behind and stored as unnecessary fat or weight gain. All foods will be digested and metabolized as needed in the most efficient way possible.

This is not a book about treating or preventing any disease; however if you or a loved one is managing Type 2 diabetes this strategy offers hope. The idea is that smaller, more frequent meals help manage hunger and control blood sugar.

Most medical professionals will agree that going long periods of time without food or eating a large meal at one time doesn't help control weight or blood sugar. Even though some research suggests there aren't any metabolic advantages to splitting calories up into smaller meals, I still highly encourage it and live by this mindset daily.

As a registered dietitian, I am most interested in this approach's ability to stabilize blood sugar which does offers health advantages. Science does show that after about 3 hours without food, blood sugar begins to fall. It takes around 4 hours for the last meal eaten to be digested, and by 5 hours post meal blood sugar can drop significantly.

For these reason, I promote a scheduled dietary routine that divides and conquers eating every 3-4 hours to help with weight loss, maintenance, and controlling hunger. This strategy starts with breakfast within 90 minutes of waking. Breakfast is arguably the most important meal of our day, but it is the most skipped.

Whether an adult or child, eating a morning meal improves our mood, sharpens our mind and prevents hunger before lunch.

Breakfast promotes less calorie intake. A satisfying, high protein breakfast can keep you feeling fuller longer. A study found that people who had eggs for breakfast ate 250 fewer calories the rest of the day. While I am pro-eggs, protein can also be found in Greek yogurt, nut butters, seeds, or smoothies. There will be breakfast examples later on.

Provides mid-morning energy. When you skip breakfast or eat one high in sugar or low in total calories, you can hit a mental wall way before lunch. I get that it can be scary eating a larger breakfast, you have the whole day to ration calories, right? Wrong! Don't worry about eating too much; experts say 20-25 percent of your total day's calories should come from breakfast; I agree! That means a minimum of 300 -500 nutrition packed calories every morning!

Promotes weight loss maintenance. The University of Massachusetts looked at those who had the healthy habit of breakfast and found people who don't eat in the morning are 4.5 times more likely to be obese than those who do. It's simple, breakfast kick-starts your metabolism and sets the stage for your day. Please have a balanced morning meal within 90 minutes of waking!

* * *

Dividing and conquering isn't the only trick to making this theory work optimally. What you eat matters, too! This book and my five food solutions are not geared to give you a list of foods not to eat. I truly believe all foods can fit and there is a time and place for even the greasiest, cheesiest, or sweetest treats imaginable. I am a huge proponent of quality foods, first and most often. If you are looking for a plan that allows you to keep highly processed factory foods, then this book is not for you.

Why quality over quantity of food matters. It may surprise you but an empty stomach does not trigger the hunger drive. The efficient and active digestion and absorption of nutrients from food does. Here is a bare-bones explanation of how digestion works.

We eat food. Our stomach breaks it down into the macronutrients; proteins, fats and carbohydrates. Next, food enters the small intestines and is further broken down into vitamins and minerals.

Then the small intestines allows the nutrients to be absorbed into the bloodstream and sent to the liver where they will be stored or sent to other parts of the body. What's left is sent to the large intestine where the remaining water is absorbed from the food and then compounded into solid waste to be expelled from the body.

Meanwhile, the nourishment that passed through the small intestine into the blood stream is busy nourishing the body. As absorption is accomplished blood-sugar levels drop and send a signal to the brain.

The red-alert is triggered that food is needed. At last, it is blood sugar dropping, not the empty stomach that signals hunger. Stabilize your blood sugar and delay hunger.

Bottom line, the more nutrient dense a food is the more nutrition available to be delivered throughout the body. You can stay well nourished, full, and satisfied on fewer calories. Calories from processed foods deliver little nutrition and the body will continue the hunger cycle until it attains the nutrients it desires. Junk food gives your large intestines a workout since little is absorbed in the small intestines for any good use. It's best to choose packaged items with legible ingredients; or better yet eat whole foods (fruits, vegetables, whole grains, lean meats, seafood, nuts, seeds and low-fat dairy foods) the way nature intended in whole form.

I'd like to explain how divide and conquer means more than just divining up total calories. As we just learned the source matters, but the combination of wholesome nutrients at each meal matters, too. Your body metabolizes and stores each of the three macronutrients (proteins, carbohydrates, and fats) very differently. In other words, your body will digest and store a 500-calorie plate of pasta very different than a plate of 500-calorie vegetables.

Another dieting myth is that a calorie is a calorie and as long as calories in versus calories out match, you're okay. Each food group offers specific benefits that the other can't do as well. That is why a balance of nutrients ensures that you are getting in the best more well trained workers your factory needs at every station. The two nutrients I feel are eaten the most out of balance are proteins and carbohydrates.

Often carbohydrates are thought about first for good reasons but protein has a significant role also and is often underutilized. Proteins include lean meats, poultry, fish, seafood, eggs, milk, yogurt, and cheese along with nuts, seeds, beans, soy, and some grains.

Among the major macronutrients, protein is the only nutrient capable of repairing, creating, or preserving muscle mass. It is simple; if you don't eat quality protein you can't have quality muscle.

Regardless of age or fitness level, building and maintaining muscle mass should be a priority. Why? Because lean muscle is the furnace is which calories are burned and energy is stored.

Without adequate muscle weight loss or maintenance fatigue or exhaustion is inevitable. Studies show that we lose ½ to 1 percent of muscle mass each year, starting in our thirties! Good nutrition and exercise can help preserve vital muscle mass.

Eat a variety of protein rich foods each day like seafood, nuts and beans, as well as lean meat, poultry, low-fat dairy and eggs. Emerging research suggests a consistent amount of about 30 grams of protein at each mealtimes is optimal. More is never better with any nutrient' excess leads to fat storage.

The underutilization of this powerful and essential nutrient is found in the notion that a consistent amount of about 30 grams of protein at mealtime is ideal. Again, this basic recommendation is for the masses, 25-35 grams is a healthy range to aim for.

My argument isn't that the majority of Americans aren't getting enough protein within the day; I'd actually argue we eat too much as a whole nation. Sounds contradicting, I know!

My argument is that we are not eating the most wholesome forms in the most efficient ways. Some reading this will be awakened that they are not eating enough protein throughout the day; others will realize they are eating too much and should scale back allowing for other foods to fill the plate. Either way, many are not eating their protein sources optimally for their wellness goals.

Here is an example of how to scale meals throughout the day.

Breakfast: Oatmeal with fruit = 6 grams of protein

Lunch: Turkey Sandwich with baked chips = 20 grams of protein

Snack: Banana = 0 grams of protein

Dinner: Steak, potato, and salad = 65 grams of protein

The problem with this menu is that there are opportunities lost to take full advantage of protein's muscle repairing and building abilities at breakfast, lunch, and snack. At dinner there is an excess consumption of protein and the grams over what the body can absorb and will either be burned as energy or stored as fat.

The take away message is to divide and conquer your

dietary protein intake with a goal of 25-35 grams at mealtime and 10-20 grams at snacks.

To do this without adding extra calories that cause unwanted weight gain, you will have to rearrange or decrease the other components of your meal. This is addressed later.

Remember, the 30 gram protein mark is the optimal amount. Do your best to meet it as often as possible. Breakfast will be your biggest challenge but not impossible. I'm not trying to get you obsessing over grams and ounces.

As long as you make a conscious choice to have a protein rich food at every meal and snack in its proper portion size, you'll be fine. From now on, ask yourself, "Where is my protein?" first when planning a menu, fixing a plate, or ordering at a restaurant.

Up next is carbohydrates, everyone's' favorite food group. Research is undisputed that nobody can afford to totally skip carbohydrates. Our bodies require, crave, and demand carbs to work effectively.

Carbohydrates are the primary energy source best suited to fuel your daily activities and exercise. Plus, it maintains blood glucose, spares protein so it can build and repair muscle tissue, and keeps the brain working at full throttle. Carbohydrates are required daily for optimal health, period.

Carbohydrates include grains, pasta, bread, crackers, cereals, fresh fruit, frozen fruit, dried fruit, and fruit juice, potatoes of all varieties, green peas, beans, corn, winter squash, and fluid milk.

The controversy isn't whether carbohydrates are needed but rather what kind and how much. The truth is one can successfully sustain health and wellness without ever eating bread, pasta, or a grain of any kind as long as fruits and starchy vegetables provide the necessary carbohydrates. And for those with specific food sensitivity or diagnosed with Celiac Disease it is a reality not a choice to avoid certain grains and traditional breads and pasta.

But let's face it, the majority of the population enjoys those foods and shouldn't feel they must forgo them in order to weigh less or be healthier.

The trick is in respecting portion sizes and understanding the metabolic mechanics behind carbohydrate digestion and absorption.

Here is a basic but revealing analogy of how carbohydrates are digested, absorbed, and stored.

Carbs begin to digest in the mouth, where enzymes in saliva start breaking it down into simpler sugars. Once the simple sugar has moved through the stomach, to the small intestines, and absorbed into the blood stream the pancreas is signaled to release a surge of insulin.

Think of insulin as your "sugar train" whose job is to go throughout the blood and pick up excess "sugar passengers." Over time, if the train never leaves the station or there are more passengers than available seats, one may develop Type 2 diabetes.

Once on the train, insulin transports the sugar to the liver where it is converted into glycogen (muscle energy). When working properly, the liver keeps a small amount and sends the rest to the brain and to the muscles.

Imagine your muscles are a kitchen sponge meant for soaking up fluid. Two conditions regulate the amount of fluid a sponge can hold—size and saturation. Visualize the glycogen as fluid being poured into a spongy muscle. Depending on how much muscle mass is available and how much glycogen is currently stored determines how much more it can soak up from the previous meal.

Here is the Ah Ha! moment. If muscles are unable to absorb and store the glycogen at hand one has approximately two precious hours to burn the remaining aerobically or it can be stored as fat! This isn't suggesting avoiding carbohydrate intake; this scene describes what happens when eaten in abundance. The extra dinner roll, second helping, mindless snacks, or the multiple sugary beverages that was never needed to start with causes the trouble.

This is exactly why nutrition professionals encourage smaller meals throughout the day. My suggestion is to divide and conquer each day. To sustain energy, muscles (sponges) should always be filled but never overflowing. By eating throughout the day in a balanced way you fill them up, and then allow some energy to be used through daily activity or exercise making room to store more with the next meal or snack and avoid the dreaded overflow.

Finding a carbohydrate "sweet spot," pun intended, can be tricky if not working with a registered dietitian who can evaluate the situation and make a sound recommendation. In general, on days when exercise is moderate in effort and last less than an hour women should consume a minimum one carbohydrate serving per meal and snack and men should consume two carbohydrate servings per meal and one to two carbohydrate per snack.

To evaluate a "sweet spot" for carbohydrate intake note how you feel. Do you feel fatigued, weak, or experience unexplained low energy throughout the day? Are you unexplainably sluggish during workouts?

Yes to these questions indicate you need to up your carbohydrate intake evenly throughout the day. Do this slowly by adding a half to a whole extra serving at each meal until improvement is noted.

No to these questions along with little to no weight loss (if desired) then you may need to decrease intake evenly through the day. Gradually remove a half to a whole serving at a time.

If you are consuming less than one serving per meal or snack look at other places calories can be decreased or increase exercise intensity. Never remove carbohydrates entirely from your daily diet to speed up weight loss.

If you answer no to these questions and are losing or maintaining the weight desired then you have found your "sweet spot!" From now on, ask yourself, "Where is my carbohydrate and how many servings are there in this meal?" when planning a menu, fixing a plate, or ordering at a restaurant.

Now it's time to talk fats. Dietary fat has been feared since the low-fat craze of the 80's. People and manufacturers went to great lengths to reduce and remove fat from their diets and products. Often fat was replaced with sugar or salt to make those foods taste good. This mindset did not solve our obesity or heart disease problem;

in fact, it only made things worse.

Fat is necessary for sustaining life. It's true. Dietary fat is critical for the overall maintenance of our bodies. The truth is that fat acts as a hunger suppressor, transports vitamins (A, D, E and K) and protects vital organs. Did you know our brains are made up of 60 percent fat? To function optimally, our brains need to maintain this level of fat. A lower amount of fat, in fact, can lead to neurological disorders.

You need a healthy dose of dietary fat daily. No more fat-phobia. Like all foods there are healthier choices and portion control is essential. Here is the fat break down.

Many wholesome foods including animal products and plants are rich in dietary fat and have unique nutritional values.

Oils are not a food group, but they provide essential fatty acids (Omega 3, 6, and 9) and originate from many different plants and some fish.

Think plants first when choosing a dietary fat source. Avocados, olives, nuts, seeds, and oils from plants do not contain any cholesterol or trans-fats that are linked to heart disease.

Animal products such as butter, shortening, bacon, egg yolks and cheese do contain cholesterol. But before you ditch these foods altogether research shows moderate intake of dietary cholesterol doesn't have as significant effect on heart disease as previously suspected. It seems trans-fats are the biggest culprit in heart disease.

Trans-fats are created through a process called hydrogenation, which makes the oil less likely to spoil.

Manufactures can keep foods on a shelf longer when using trans-fats. But enough science has touted trans-fat as deadly and US cities, including New York and Philadelphia, as well as some European countries, such as Denmark and Switzerland have placed bans on this substance.

Hopefully you are ready to avoid and remove trans-fats from your diet. Start by looking at the ingredient list for the words "partially hydrogenated" vegetable oil, another term for trans-fat.

Don't rely on the terms "trans-fat free" or 0 grams trans-fat on the nutrition label. In the U.S. if a food has less than 0.5 grams of trans fat per serving, the food label can read 0 grams trans-fat. Sounds insignificant, but if you eat multiple servings of foods with 0.5 grams of trans-fat, you could exceed recommended limits.

Now that you are aware of which dietary fats to choose and avoid, you probably are wondering how much should you eat?

Learning how much dietary fat to intake to achieve an ideal weight and obtain optimal health takes time if not working with a registered dietitian who can evaluate the situation and make a sound recommendation.

In general, on days when exercise is moderate in exertion and lasts less than one hour women should consume at minimum one fat serving per meal and men should consume two fat servings per meal.

To evaluate intake note how you feel. Are you full and satisfied after meals? Do you get hungry within two hours of finishing a meal?

If you are not satisfied after completing a meal or get hungry within 2 hours of ending a meal, then you may not be eating enough fat to suppress hunger. Increase dietary fat intake at each meal. Add one whole extra serving at a time until improvement is noted.

Feeling full and satisfied after a meal for up to 3-4 hours is a good sign your meal is well balanced and includes enough dietary fat. If little or no weight loss (if desired) is not happening then examine all portion sizes in the meal first before eliminating fat servings.

Use common sense when preparing food and save fried, heavily sautéed, bacon, lard, and cream sauces for special occasions. Limit red meats (beef, pork, or egg yolks) to no more than once daily. Check your cholesterol annually by a doctor and seek advice from a health professional if your cholesterol needs to be lowered.

From now on, ask yourself, "Where is my fat choice and how many are there in this meal?" when planning a menu, fixing a plate, or ordering at a restaurant.

The body can only process and utilize so many nutrients in a 3-4 hour period of time. Our job is to give it the most high quality nutrients possible every 3-4 hours to keep it up and running seamlessly. The body can't overwork itself, it can only store extra. It doesn't want to under work either, it will just get sick, slow down your metabolism, and become fatigued.

The purpose of this strategy is to become aware of the areas you need to improve, and do your best. Naturally, you will begin to eat smaller meals because you will be less hungry once you divide and conquer your day. The easiest way to start becoming aware of the timing is to set an alarm on your phone for 3.5 hours. This begins the awareness process, which is a crucial first step to change.

Chapter 12

More Matters

And God said, "Behold, I have given you every plant yielding seed that is on the face of all the earth, and every tree with seed in its fruit. You shall have them for food."—Genesis 1:29 (ESV)

My third food solution for better health is my personal favorite. Not only does it encourage the food group the Western world lacks the most, but it packs the most powerful potential to prevent chronic disease, increase longevity, and help you maintain a healthy weight.

Food solution number three is committing to a fruit or vegetable serving or both at every meal and snack.

It is well-documented that eating fruits and vegetables may reduce the risk of many diseases. In fact, the Dietary Guidelines for Americans recommends eating more fruits and vegetables than any other food group. Actually, they endorse half your plate being filled with fruits and vegetables at every meal.

You've probably heard that plant-based foods pack potent phytochemicals, polyphenols, and antioxidants. But, do you know what these terms mean?

Phytochemicals are found in plant foods such as fruits, vegetables, beans, and whole grains. Other common names for phytochemicals are antioxidants, flavonoids, phytonutrients, flavones, isofalvones, catchins, and polyphenols.

Basically, phytochemicals do a really good job at fighting disease and boosting our immune system. Think of your immune system as your own secret service, hidden out of sight, but there to jump to your defense against germs and other nasty invaders. We want to keep our immune systems as strong as possible. The president doesn't want weak bodyguards and neither do you!

There's no question that eating three to five servings of fruits and vegetables daily will improve your health. But more experts are saying healthy eating is not only about how many servings you eat.

It's about the variety you pick, too. Maintaining an eating pattern that includes a variety of fruits and vegetables will provide your body with a wide assortment of all the beneficial compounds. While you're choosing your plant based choice at every meal and snack make sure there is a variety in color and texture, too.

There are two types of vegetables, starchy and non-starchy. Starchy vegetables like potatoes, corn, beans, and peas contain significantly more carbohydrates and calories per serving. *A complete list is located at the end of the chapter.* Some diet approaches get wrapped up in glycemic index and labeling certain fruits or vegetables as "bad" or encouraging only half a banana at a time.

While there is good science backing the glycemic index, it is irrelevant if you stick to wholefoods that have been low-to-no processed; which is exactly what I preach from the nutrition mountain tops!

For those not tainted by the glycemic index (GI) mindset, let me explain it. The glycemic index is a measure of how quickly foods containing carbohydrates, such as fruits, potatoes, cereals, and baked goods raise glucose (sugar) levels in the body's bloodstream. If a food causes a sudden and sharp spike in blood sugar levels after two hours of ingestion it is said to have a high glycemic index.

Those foods are typically recommended to be avoided: white bread, sugar, pasta, and bananas to name a few. When the opposite happens and there is less of an effect on blood sugar, it is deemed a low GI food.

While I completely agree we should lessen our intake of white flour and sugar, I will stand in defense of white potatoes because most individuals don't eat large quantities of these foods by themselves in one sitting.

It is true that eating foods rich in carbohydrates all by themselves will not leave someone full and satisfied for every long, but there are other ways of going about choosing meals and snacks without ranking any fruit or vegetables as bad or off limits.

From here on out free the white potato, bananas, carrots and others from their GI labels and focus on learning how to apply the third food solution into your daily diets. There is nothing bad about starchy vegetables or fruits, my first request will be become aware that they are not the ONLY type of plant you are eating.

Non-starchy vegetables get the golden halo and include dark leafy greens, broccoli, cauliflower, carrots, green beans, asparagus, mushrooms, and summer squash etc. *A complete list is located at the end of the chapter.* Even though these foods pack the most phytonutrient punch, they tend to be the least glamorous food group that generates the most resistance. But they are the only group that no portion control is needed and more is better!

Vegetables are full of vitamins, minerals, fiber, and phytochemicals (disease fighters) and offer so few calories that the serving size is literally up to you. Seriously, there is only 7 calories in a cup of raw-spinach and roughly 30 calories in a cup of chopped broccoli.

Plant-based foods including starchy and non-starchy vegetables are the most high quality factory workers you can employ (nutrients) and they are not hired (eaten) nearly enough to serve us daily. Enjoy fresh, frozen, or canned in water. Bake, boil, microwave, grill, sauté, steam, or eat them raw just make sure you eat them often.

Fruit in any form typically doesn't need convincing to be eaten, but we still either don't make a conscious choice to eat enough, or we eat way too much in one meal. Both are not the best strategy for health or wellness.

Enjoy fresh, frozen, or canned in water or natural juices. None are significantly better than the other, and every type of fruit has its place in the diet. I actually buy fresh, frozen, and canned most weeks for different reasons. Canned fruit can be a great money and time saver.

I hear this often, "Fresh fruits and vegetables are better for you than canned or frozen because the processing removes all the nutrients."

Let me assure this not necessarily true and that incorporating a variety of fresh, frozen, and canned produce into your weekly menus will better help you meet serving recommendations and save some time and money in the process.

You can feel confident that the nutrient content of canned and frozen fruits and vegetables is comparable to fresh and, in some instances; it could be higher than fresh. The positive of fresh and frozen is that is processed immediately after harvesting, so nutrient losses after picking are minimal.

Sure the canning or freezing process may cause some loss of nutrients, but so does the packaging, shipping, and purchasing then waiting on the counter to be consumed of the fresh varieties.

While I am a huge fan and proponent of visiting your local farmer's markets, I also keep frozen and canned fruits and vegetables in my own pantry. They are more economical choices and great as backups when you don't have time to make to the store or market.

My best advice is your diet should include a variety of fruits and vegetables. Choosing canned and frozen forms of fruits and vegetables increase the variety and add interest to meals and snacks. Don't be afraid to explore the frozen and canned aisle at the supermarket.

When you do purchase fresh produce make sure you probably store it at home. Nothing is sadder than having to toss spoiled food. A simple trick with any perishable food is to remember the FIFO rule: First In, First Out. Use the oldest first and continually rotate foods to ensure freshness while reducing waste. The FIFO rule applies to every type of food- fresh, frozen, canned, and dried.

Here is a simple guide to storage from Fruits and Veggies More Matters dot org:

Fresh
- Use within a few days.
- Some can be left at room temperature to ripen, and then refrigerated.

Frozen
- Store at 0 degrees F or less.
- Use before the "use by" date on the package.
- As a rule, use within 6 months.

Canned
- Check the "use by" date on the can.
- Most canned goods have a shelf life of about 2 years.
- Store at room temperature (about 75 degrees F).

Dried
- Store in a cool, dark place (warmth makes the food spoil faster).
- Some dried foods may be refrigerated- check the package.
- Most will last from 4 months to a year.

It's silly that storing fresh produce could be so complicated! But, always place fruits and vegetables in separated, perforated plastic bags with a paper towel to help reduce moisture.

Never store fruits in the same draw as vegetables. Fruits produce ethylene that can negatively affect vegetables.

Foods to store in your refrigerator:
- Apples
- Aprictos
- Asian pears
- Berries
- Cherries
- Cut Fruit
- Figs
- Grapes
- Artichokes
- Asparagus
- Green Beans
- Beets
- Belgian Endive
- Broccoli
- Brussel Sprouts
- Cabbage
- Carrots
- Cauliflower
- Celery
- Cut Vegetables
- Green Onions
- Herbs (not basil)
- Leafy Greens

- Leeks
- Lettuce
- Mushrooms
- Peas
- Radishes
- Spinach
- Sprouts
- Summer Squashes
- Sweet Corn

Not all produce needs to go straight to the refrigerator and should have time to ripen on the counter first. Let these items ripen, then store in the refrigerator.

- Avocados
- Kiwi
- Nectarines
- Peaches
- Pears
- Plums
- Plumcots

There are some items that should only be stored at room temperature for best flavor and texture. Refrigeration of the following foods can cause cold damage or prevent them from fully ripening and you will miss out on the best taste possible. Lastly, I know a fruit bowl is pretty décor, but truthfully these foods should be stored away from direct sunlight and in a well-ventilated area in your pantry.

- Apples
- Bananas
- Citrus Fruits
- Mangoes
- Melons
- Papayas
- Persimmons
- Pinapple
- Plantain
- Pomegrantaes
- Basil
- Cucumber
- Eggplant
- Garlic
- Ginger
- Onions
- Peppers
- Potatoes
- Pumpkins
- Sweet Potatoes
- Tomatoes
- Winter Squashes

As if you weren't already overwhelmed by all the instructions to just get fresh produce into your homes and bellies, there is a final small but significant step—cleaning. As a reminder, never store your produce near or with raw meat, poultry, and seafood.

No one wants dirt or grim on their produce so washing it makes good sense. But, never use detergent or bleach to wash any food. Simply rinse produce under running tap water prior to use versus as soon as you get home with it. Washing too far in advance may remove some of the natural preservatives that help keep it fresh longer. Except for heads of lettuce and leafy greens that defy the rule and will remain crisper when washed right away, wrapped in a paper towel and refrigerated.

Those foods with skins and rinds need to be washed and dried before cutting or peeling. Packaged fruits and vegetables labeled "ready-to-eat," "washed', or "triple wash" do not require any additional washing.

This is the first food solution that focuses on what to eat, but notice I am not dictating what you cannot eat. So, I won't harp on what fruit or vegetable you choose, I'm just begging that you choose a source of one or both at every meal and snack within the proper portion size. Portion control even with the healthiest of foods is essential for weight maintenance. Here is a quick reference of the most popular produce:

Starchy Vegetables
Corn, on cob - 1 large
Corn, cooked - ½ cup
Mixed Vegetables - 1 cup
Potato, baked - medium
Potato, boiled - ½ cup
Potato, mashed - ½ cup
Squash, winter - ½ cup

Yam, sweet potato - med
yam, sweet potato - ½ cup
Baked Beans, cooked - ½ c
Beans, canned - ½ cup
Lentils, cooked - ½ cup
Peas, cooked - ½ cup
Refried beans - ½ cup

Fruit
Fresh, whole - 1 medium
Fresh or Frozen, cubed- 1 c
Fresh, juiced - 1 cup
Canned, unsweet- ½ cup
Dried fruit - ¼ cup

Non- starchy Vegetables
Unlimited Serving Size!!
Salad Greens (All Varieties)
Amaranth
Artichoke
Artichoke Hearts
Asparagus
Baby Corn (typically pickled)
Bamboo shoots
Bean Sprouts
Beans, Green, French Style
Beets
Broccoli
Brussels Sprouts
Cabbage, (green, bok choy)

Carrots
Cauliflower
Celery
Chayote
Coleslaw, no dressing
Cucumber
Daikon
Eggplant
Gourds (bitter, bottle, luffa)
Green onions or scallions
Greens -collard,kale,mustard
Hearts of palm
Leeks
Mixed Vegs (no corn, pasta)
Mung Bean Sprouts
Mushrooms, all kinds, fresh
Okra
onions
Pea Pods
Peppers (all varieties)
Radishes
Rutabaga
Sauerkraut
Soybean sprouts
Spinach
Squash (summer, zucchini)
Sugar Snap Peas
Swiss Chard
Tomato
Tomatoes, canned

Tomato sauce
Tomato / veg juice - 1 cup
Turnips
Water chestnuts
Yard - Long Beans

As I close out the chapter on eating your fruits and vegetables, I can't leave without making a strong case for getting involved and visiting your local farmer's market. I understand it is more expensive, usually inconvenient, and not available to everyone everywhere. That's ok. Just ponder the potential.

Entrepreneurship fuels America's economic innovation and prosperity, and it can be debated that the farmer was one of the original entrepreneurs.

Often located off the beaten path, farm families are still considered locally owned businesses that help build strong communities by linking neighbors in economic and social relationships, plus regularly giving back to local causes. Like any passionate business owner, farmers take pride in their product and get shear satisfaction from happy customers.

I look at supporting our local Farmer's Markets as a win-win that can't be beat. Farmer's markets offer the farmer a storefront, a centralized spot to showcase their farm-fresh foods.

From persimmons to peaches, from bok choy to butter beans, local Farmer's Markets are the one place to go for the freshest fruits and vegetables that are grown in the rich soil across our great country.